MW01675063

SOUS VIDE COOKBOOK 2022

RECIPES FOR BEGINNERS

MICK FORTIS

Table of Contents

Chicken Stock

Prep + Cook Time: 12 hours 25 minutes | Servings: 3

Ingredients:

2 lb chicken, any parts – thighs, breasts

5 cups water

2 celery sticks, chopped

2 white onions, chopped

Directions:

Make a water bath, place Sous Vide in it, and set to 194 F. Separate all the ingredients in 2 vacuum bags, fold the top of the bags 2-3 times. Place in the water bath. Set the timer for 12 hours.

Once the timer has stopped, remove the bags and transfer the ingredients to a pot. Boil the ingredients over high heat for 10 minutes. Turn off heat and strain. Use the stock as a soup base.

Onion Pomodoro Sauce

Prep + Cook Time: 30 minutes | Servings: 4

Ingredients

4 cups tomatoes, halved and cored

½ onion, chopped

½ tsp sugar

¼ cup fresh oregano

2 garlic cloves, minced

Salt and black pepper to taste

5 tbsp olive oil

Directions:

Prepare a water bath and place the Sous Vide in it. Set to 175 F. Place the tomatoes, oregano, garlic, onion and sugar in a vacuum-sealable bag. Release air by the water displacement method, seal and submerge the bag in the water bath. Cook for 15 minutes.

Once the timer has stopped, remove the bag and transfer the content into a blender and mix for 1 minute until smooth. Top with black pepper.

Bell Pepper Puree

Prep + Cook Time: 40 minutes | Servings: 4

Ingredients:

8 red bell peppers, cored

⅓ cup olive oil

2 tbsp lemon juice

3 cloves garlic, crushed

2 tsp sweet paprika

Directions:

Make a water bath and place Sous Vide in it and set to 183 F. Put the bell peppers, garlic, and olive oil in a vacuum-sealable bag. Release air by the water displacement method, seal and submerge the bags in the water bath. Set the timer for 20 minutes and cook.

Once the timer has stopped, remove the bag and unseal. Transfer the bell pepper and garlic to a blender and puree to smooth. Place a pan over medium heat; add bell pepper puree and the remaining ingredients. Cook for 3 minutes. Serve warm or cold as a dip.

Jalapeno Seasoning

Prep + Cook Time: 70 minutes | Servings: 6

Ingredients:

2 jalapeno peppers

2 green chili peppers

2 cloves garlic, crushed

1 onion, peeled only

3 tsp oregano powder

3 tsp black pepper powder

2 tsp rosemary powder

10 tsp aniseed powder

Directions

Make a water bath, place Sous Vide in it, and set to 185 F. Place the peppers and onion in a vacuum-sealable bag. Release air by the water displacement method, seal and submerge the bag in the water bath. Set the timer for 40 minutes.

Once the timer has stopped, remove and unseal the bag. Transfer the pepper and onion with 2 tablespoons of water to a blender and puree to smooth.

Place a pot over low heat, add in pepper puree and the remaining ingredients. Simmer for 15 minutes. Turn off heat and cool. Store in a spice jar, refrigerate, and use for up to 7 days. Use it as a spice.

Beef Broth

Prep + Cook Time: 13 hours 25 minutes | Servings: 6

Ingredients:

3 lb beef feet

1 ½ lb beef bones

½ lb grounded beef

5 cups tomato paste

6 sweet onions

3 heads garlic

6 tbsp black pepper

5 sprigs thyme

4 bay leaves

10 cups water

Directions:

Preheat an oven to 425 F. Place beef bones and beef feet in a roasting pan and rub them with the tomato paste. Add garlic and onion. Set aside. Place and crumble ground beef in another roasting pan. Place the roasting pans in the oven and roast until dark brown.

Once done, drain fat from the roasting pans. Make a water bath in a large container, place Sous Vide in it, and set to 195 F. Separate the ground beef, roasted vegetables, black pepper, thyme, and bay leaves in 3 vacuum bags. Deglaze the roasting pans with water and add it to the bags. Fold the top of the bags 2 to 3 times.

Place the bags in the water bath and clip it to the Sous Vide container. Set the timer for 13 hours. Once the timer has stopped, remove the bags and transfer the ingredients to a pot. Bring the ingredients to a boil over high heat. Cook for 15 minutes. Turn off heat and strain. Use the stock as a soup base.

Garlic Basil Rub

Prep + Cook Time: 55 minutes | Servings: 15

Ingredients:

2 heads garlic, crushed

2 tsp olive oil

A pinch salt

1 head fennel bulb, chopped

2 lemons, zested and juiced

¼ sugar

25 basil leaves

Directions:

Make a water bath, place Sous Vide in it, and set to 185 F. Place the fennel and sugar in a vacuum-sealable bag. Release air by the water displacement method, seal and submerge the bag in the water bath. Set the timer for 40 minutes.Once the timer has stopped, remove and unseal the bag.

Transfer the fennel, sugar, and remaining listed ingredients to a blender and puree to smooth. Store in a spice container and use up to a week with refrigeration.

Honey & Onion Balsamic Dressing

Prep + Cook Time: 1 hour 55 minutes | Servings: 1)

Ingredients

3 sweet onions, chopped

1 tbsp butter

Salt and black pepper to taste

2 tbsp balsamic vinegar

1 tbsp honey

2 tsp of fresh thyme leaves

Directions

Prepare a water bath and place the Sous Vide in it. Set to 186 F.

Heat a skillet over medium heat with butter. Add onions, season with salt and pepper and cook for 10 minutes. Add in balsamic vinegar and cook for 1 minute. Remove from the heat and pour in honey.

Place the mix in a vacuum-sealable bag. Release air by the water displacement method, seal and submerge the bag in the water bath. Cook for 90 minutes. Once the timer has stopped, remove the bag and transfer to a platter. Garnish with fresh thyme. Serve with pizza or sandwich.

Tomato Sauce

Prep + Cook Time: 55 minutes | Servings: 4

Ingredients:

1 (16-oz) can tomatoes, crushed

1 small white onion, diced

1 cup fresh basil leaves

1 tbsp olive oil

1 clove garlic, crushed

Salt to taste

1 bay leaf

1 red chili

Directions:

Make a water bath, place Sous Vide in it, and set to 185 F. Place all the listed ingredients in a vacuum-sealable bag. Release air by the water displacement method, seal and submerge the bag in the water bath. Set the timer for 40 minutes. Once the timer has stopped, remove and unseal the bag. Discard the bay leaf and transfer the remaining ingredients to a blender and puree smooth.Serve as a side sauce.

Seafood Stock

Prep + Cook Time: 10 hours 10 minutes | Servings: 6

Ingredients:

1 lb shrimp shells, with heads and tails

3 cups water

1 tbsp olive oil

2 tsp salt

2 sprigs rosemary

½ head garlic, crushed

½ cup celery leaves, chopped

Directions:

Make a water bath, place Sous Vide in it, and set to 180 F. Toss the shrimp with the olive oil. Place the shrimp with the remaining listed ingredients in a vacuum-sealable bag. Release air, seal and submerge the bag into the water bath, and set the timer for 10 hours.

Fish Broth

Prep + Cook Time: 10 hours 15 minutes | Servings: 4

Ingredients:

5 cups water

½ lb fish fillets, skin

1 lb fish head

5 medium green onions

3 sweet onion

¼ lb black seaweed (Kombu)

Directions:

Make a water bath, place Sous Vide in it, and set to 194 F. Separate all the listed ingredients equally into 2 vacuum bags, fold the top of the bags 2 times. Place them in the water bath and clip it to the Sous Vide container. Set the timer for 10 hours.

Once the timer has stopped, remove the bags and transfer the ingredients to a pot. Boil the ingredients over high heat for 5 minutes Turn off heat and strain. Refrigerate and use for up to 14 days.

Mustard Asparagus Dressing

Prep + Cook Time: 30 minutes | Servings: 2

Ingredients

1 Bunch large asparagus

Salt and black pepper to taste

¼ cup olive oil

1 tsp Dijon mustard

1 tsp dill

1 tsp red wine vinegar

1 hard-boiled egg, chopped

Fresh parsley, chopped

Directions

Prepare a water bath and place the Sous Vide in it. Set to 186 F.

Chop the bottom of the asparagus and discard it.

Peel the bottom of the stalk and place in a vacuum-sealable bag. Release air by the water displacement method, seal and submerge the bag in the water bath. Cook for 15 minutes.

Once the timer has stopped, remove the bag and transfer to an ice bath. Separate the cooking juices. In a bowl, for the vinaigrette, combine olive oil, vinegar and mustard; stir well. Season with salt and move it to a mason jar. Seal and shake until well combined. Top with parsley, egg and the vinaigrette.

Vegetable Stock

Prep + Cook Time: 12 hours 35 minutes | Servings: 10)

Ingredients:

1 ½ cups celery root, diced

1 ½ cups leeks, diced

½ cup fennel bulb, diced

4 cloves garlic, crushed

1 tbsp olive oil

6 cups water

1 ½ cups mushrooms

½ cup parsley, chopped

1 tbsp black peppercorns

1 bay leaf

Directions:

Make a water bath, place Sous Vide in it, and set to 180 F. Preheat an oven to 450 F. Place the leeks, celery, fennel, garlic, and olive oil in a bowl. Toss them. Transfer to a roasting pan and tuck them in the oven. Roast for 20 minutes.

Place the roasted vegetables with its juices, water, parsley, peppercorns, mushrooms, and bay leaf in a vacuum-sealable bag.

Release air, seal and submerge the bag into the water bath and set the timer for 12 hours. Cover the water bath's container with a plastic wrap to reduce evaporation and keep adding water to the bath to keep the vegetables covered.

Once the timer has stopped, remove and unseal the bag. Strain the ingredients. Cool and use frozen for up to 1 month.

Once the timer has stopped, remove and unseal the bag. Strain the ingredients. Cool and use frozen for up to 2 weeks.

Garlic Tabasco Edamame Cheese

Prep + Cook Time: 1 hour 6 minutes | Servings: 4

Ingredients

1 tbsp olive oil

4 cups fresh edamame in pods

1 tsp salt

1 garlic clove, minced

1 tbsp red pepper flakes

1 tbsp Tabasco sauce

Directions

Prepare a water bath and place the Sous Vide in it. Set to 186 F.

Heat a pot with water over high heat and blanch the edamame pots for 60 seconds. Strain them and transfer into an ice water bath. Combine the garlic, red pepper flakes, Tabasco sauce, and olive oil.

Place the edamame in a vacuum-sealable bag. Pour the Tabasco sauce. Release air by the water displacement method, seal and submerge the bag in the water bath. Cook for 1 hour. Once the timer has stopped, remove the bag and transfer into a bowl and serve.

Herby Mashed Snow Peas

Prep + Cook Time: 55 minutes | Servings: 6

Ingredients

½ cup vegetable broth

1 pound fresh snow peas

Zest of 1 lemon

2 tbsp chopped fresh basil

1 tbsp olive oil

Salt and black pepper to taste

2 tbsp chopped fresh chives

2 tbsp chopped fresh parsley

¾ tsp garlic powder

Directions

Prepare a water bath and place the Sous Vide in it. Set to 186 F.

Combine the peas, lemon zest, basil, olive oil, black pepper, chives, parsley, salt, and garlic powder and place them in a vacuum-sealable bag. Release air by the water displacement method, seal and submerge the bag in the water bath. Cook for 45 minutes. Once the timer has stopped, remove the bag and transfer into a blender and mix well.

Sage Roasted Potato Mash

Prep + Cook Time: 1 hour 35 minutes | Servings: 6

Ingredients

¼ cup butter

12 sweet potatoes, unpeeled

10 garlic cloves, chopped

4 tsp salt

6 tbsp olive oil

5 fresh sage sprigs

1 tbsp paprika

Directions

Prepare a water bath and place the Sous Vide in it. Set to 192 F.

Combine the potatoes, garlic, salt, olive oil and 2 or 3 thyme springs and place in a vacuum-sealable bag. Release air by the water displacement method, seal and submerge the bag in the water bath. Cook for 1 hour and 15 minutes.

Preheat the oven to 450 F. Once the timer has stopped, remove the potatoes and transfer into a bowl. Separate the cooking juices.

Combine well the potatoes with butter and the remaining sage springs. Transfer into a baking tray, previously lined with aluminium foil. Make a hole in the center of the potatoes and pour the cooking juices in. Bake the potatoes for 10 minutes, turning 5 minutes later. Discard the sage. Transfer to a plate and serve sprinkled with paprika.

Buttered Asparagus with Thyme & Cheese

Prep + Cook Time: 21 minutes | Servings: 6

Ingredients

¼ cup shaved Pecorino Romano cheese

16 oz fresh asparagus, trimmed

4 tbsp butter, cubed

Salt to taste

1 garlic clove, minced

1 tbsp thyme

Directions

Prepare a water bath and place the Sous Vide in it. Set to 186 F.

Place the asparagus in a vacuum-sealable bag. Add the butter cubes, garlic, salt, and thyme. Release air by the water displacement method, seal and submerge the bag in the water bath. Cook for 14 minutes.

Once the timer has stopped, remove the bag and transfer the asparagus to a plate. Sprinkle with some cooking juices. Garnish with the Pecorino Romano cheese.

Tasty Parsnips with Honey Glaze

Prep + Cook Time: 1 hour 8 minutes | Servings: 4

Ingredients

1 pound parsnips, peeled and trimmed

3 tbsp butter

2 tbsp honey

1 tsp olive oil

Salt and black pepper to taste

1 tbsp chopped fresh parsley

Directions

Prepare a water bath and place the Sous Vide in it. Set to 186 F.

Place the parsnips, butter, honey, olive oil, salt, and pepper in a vacuum-sealable bag. Release air by the water displacement method, seal and submerge the bag in the water bath. Cook for 1 hour.

Heat a skillet over medium heat. Once the timer has stopped, remove the bag and transfer the contents into the skillet and cook for 2 minutes until the liquid turns a glaze. Add the parsley and mix quickly. Serve.

Cream of Tomatoes with Cheese Sandwich

Prep + Cook Time: 55 minutes | Servings: 8)

Ingredients

½ cup cream cheese

2 pounds tomatoes, cut into wedges

Salt and black pepper to taste

2 tbsp olive oil

2 garlic cloves, minced

½ tsp chopped fresh sage

⅛ tsp red pepper flakes

½ tsp white wine vinegar

2 tbsp butter

4 slices bread

2 slices halloumi cheese

Directions

Prepare a water bath and place the Sous Vide in it. Set to 186 F. Put the tomatoes in a colander over a bowl and season with salt. Stir well. Allow to chill for 30 minutes. Discard the juices. Combine the olive oil, garlic, sage, black pepper, salt, and pepper flakes.

Place in a vacuum-sealable bag. Release air by the water displacement method, seal and submerge the bag in the water bath. Cook for 40 minutes.

Once the timer has stopped, remove the bag and transfer into a blender. Add in vinegar and cream cheese. Mix until smooth. Transfer to a plate and season with salt and pepper if needed.

To make the cheese bars: heat a skillet over medium heat. Grease the bread slices with butter and put into the skillet. Lay cheese slices over the bread and place over another buttery bread. Toast for 1-2 minutes. Repeat with the remaining bread. Cut into cubes. Serve over the warm soup.

Maple Beet Salad with Cashews & Queso Fresco

Prep + Cook Time: 1 hour 35 minutes | Servings: 8)

Ingredients

6 large beets, peeled and cut into chunks

Salt and black pepper to taste

3 tbsp maple syrup

2 tbsp butter

Zest of 1 large orange

1 tbsp olive oil

½ tsp cayenne pepper

1½ cups cashews

6 cup arugula

3 tangerines, peeled and segmented

1 cup queso fresco, crumbled

Directions

Prepare a water bath and place the Sous Vide in it. Set to 186 F.

Place the beet chunks in a vacuum-sealable bag. Season with salt and pepper. Add 2 tbsp of maple syrup, butter, and orange zest.

Release air by the water displacement method, seal and submerge the bag in the water bath. Cook for 1 hour and 15 minutes.

Preheat the oven to 350 F.

Mix the remaining maple syrup, olive oil, salt, and cayenne. Add in cashews and stir well. Transfer the cashew mixture into a baking tray, previously lined with wax pepper and bake for 10 minutes. Set aside and allow to cool.

Once the timer has stopped, remove the beets and discard the cooking juices. Put the arugula on a serving plate, beets and tangerine wedges all over. Scatter with queso fresco and cashew mix to serve.

Cheesy Bell Peppers with Cauliflower

Prep + Cook Time: 52 minutes | Servings: 5

Ingredients

½ cup shaved Provolone cheese

1 head cauliflower, cut florets

2 garlic cloves, minced

Salt and black pepper to taste

2 tbsp butter

1 tbsp olive oil

½ large red bell pepper, cut strips

½ large yellow bell pepper, cut into strips

½ large orange bell pepper, cut into strips

Directions

Prepare a water bath and place the Sous Vide in it. Set to 186 F.

Combine well the cauliflower florets, 1 clove of garlic, salt, pepper, half of butter, and half of olive oil.

In another bowl, mix the bell peppers, remaining garlic, remaining salt, pepper, remaining butter, and remaining olive oil.

Place the cauliflower in a vacuum-sealable bag. Place the bell peppers in another vacuum-sealable bag. Release air by the water displacement method, seal and submerge the bags in the water bath. Cook for 40 minutes.

Once the timer has stopped, remove the bags and transfer the contents into a serving bowl. Discard the cooking juices. Combine the vegetables and top with Provolone cheese.

Fall Squash Cream Soup

Prep + Cook Time: 2 hours 20 minutes | Servings: 6

Ingredients

¾ cup heavy cream

1 winter squash, chopped

1 large pear

½ yellow onion, diced

3 fresh thyme sprigs

1 garlic clove, chopped

1 tsp ground cumin

Salt and black pepper to taste

4 tbsp crème fraîche

Directions

Prepare a water bath and place the Sous Vide in it. Set to 186 F.

Combine the squash, pear, onion, thyme, garlic, cumin, and salt. Place in a vacuum-sealable bag. Release air by the water displacement method, seal and submerge in water bath. Cook for 2 hours.

Once the timer has stopped, remove the bag and transfer all the contents into a blender. Puree until smooth. Add in cream and stir well. Season with salt and pepper. Transfer the mix into serving bowls and top with some créme fraiche. Garnish with pear chunks.

Celery & Leek Potato Soup

Prep + Cook Time: 2 hours 15 minutes | Servings: 8)

Ingredients

8 tbsp butter

4 red potatoes, sliced

1 yellow onion, cut into ¼-inch pieces

1 celery stalk, cut into ½-inch pieces

4 cups ½-inch diced leeks, white parts only

1 cup vegetable stock

1 carrot, chopped

4 garlic cloves, minced

2 bay leaves

Salt and black pepper to taste

2 cups heavy cream

¼ cup chopped fresh chives

Directions

Prepare a water bath and place the Sous Vide in it. Set to 186 F.

Place the potatoes, carrots, onion, celery, leeks, vegetable stock, butter, garlic, and bay leaves in a vacuum-sealable bag. Release air by the water displacement method, seal and submerge the bag in the water bath. Cook for 2 hours.

Once the timer has stopped, remove the bag and transfer into a blender. Discard the bay leaves. Mix the contents and season with salt and pepper. Pour the cream slowly and blend 2-3 minutes until smooth. Drain the contents and garnish with chives to serve.

Lemon Collard Greens Salad with Cranberries

Prep + Cook Time: 15 minutes | Servings: 6

Ingredients

6 cups fresh collard greens, stemmed

6 tbsp olive oil

2 garlic cloves, crushed

4 tbsp lemon juice

½ tsp salt

¾ cup dried cranberries

Directions

Prepare a water bath and place the Sous Vide in it. Set to 196 F. Combine the collard greens with 2 tbsp of olive oil. Place it in a vacuum-sealable bag. Release air by the water displacement method, seal and submerge the bag in the water bath. Cook for 8 minutes.

Stir the remaining olive oil, garlic, lemon juice and salt. Once the timer has stopped, remove the collard greens and transfer onto a serving plate. Sprinkle with the dressing. Garnish with cranberries.

Citrus Corn with Tomato Sauce

Prep + Cook Time: 55 minutes | Servings: 8)

Ingredients

⅓ cup olive oil

4 ears yellow corn, husked

Salt and black pepper to taste

1 large tomato, chopped

3 tbsp lemon juice

2 garlic cloves, minced

1 serrano pepper, seeded

4 scallions, green parts only, chopped

½ bunch fresh cilantro leaves, chopped

Directions

Prepare a water bath and place the Sous Vide in it. Set to 186 F. Whisk the corns with olive oil and season with salt and pepper. Place them in a vacuum-sealable bag. Release air by the water displacement method, seal and submerge the bag in the water bath. Cook for 45 minutes.

Meantime, combine well the tomato, lemon juice, garlic, serrano pepper, scallions, cilantro, and the remaining olive oil in a bowl. Preheat a grill over high heat.

Once the timer has stopped, remove the corns and transfer to the grill and cook for 2-3 minutes. Allow to cool. Cut the kernels from the cob and pour in tomato sauce. Serve with fish, salad or tortilla chips.

Ginger Tamari Brussels Sprouts with Sesame

Prep + Cook Time: 43 minutes | Servings: 6

Ingredients

1½ pounds Brussels sprouts, halved

2 garlic cloves, minced

2 tbsp vegetable oil

1 tbsp tamari sauce

1 tsp grated ginger

¼ tsp red pepper flakes

¼ tsp toasted sesame oil

1 tbsp sesame seeds

Directions

Prepare a water bath and place Sous Vide in it. Set to 186 F. Heat a pot over medium heat and combine the garlic, vegetable oil, tamari sauce, ginger, and red pepper flakes. Cook for 4-5 minutes. Set aside.

Place the brussels sprouts in a vacuum-sealable bag and pour in tamari mixture. Release air by the water displacement method, seal and submerge the bag in the water bath. Cook for 30 minutes.

Once the timer has stopped, remove the bag and pat dry with kitchen towel. Reserve the cooking juices. Transfer the sprouts to a bowl and combine with the sesame oil. Plate the sprouts and sprinkle with cooking juices. Garnish with sesame seeds.

Beet Spinach Salad

Prep + Cook Time: 2 hours 25 minutes | Servings: 3

Ingredients:

1 ¼ cup beets, trimmed and cut into bite-sized pieces

1 cup fresh spinach, chopped

2 tbsp olive oil

1 tbsp lemon juice, freshly juiced

1 tsp balsamic vinegar

2 garlic cloves, crushed

1 tbsp butter

Salt and black pepper to taste

Directions:

Rinse well and clean beets. Chop into bite-sized pieces and place in a vacuum-sealable bag along with butter and crushed garlic. Cook in Sous Vide for 2 hours at 185 F. Set aside to cool.

Boil a large pot of water and place spinach in it. Cook for one minute, and then remove from the heat. Drain well. Transfer to a vacuum-sealable bag and cook in Sous Vide for 10 minutes at 180 F. Remove from the water bath and cool completely. Place in a large bowl and add cooked beets. Season with salt, pepper, vinegar, olive oil, and lemon juice. Serve immediately.

Garlic Greens with Mint

Prep + Cook Time: 30 minutes | Servings: 2

Ingredients:

½ cup fresh chicory, torn

½ cup wild asparagus, finely chopped

½ cup Swiss chard, torn

¼ cup fresh mint, chopped

¼ cup arugula, torn

2 garlic cloves, minced

½ tsp salt

4 tbsp lemon juice, freshly squeezed

2 tbsp olive oil

Directions:

Fill a large pot with salted water and add greens. Cook for 3 minutes. Remove and drain. Gently squeeze with your hands and using a sharp knife chop the greens. Transfer to a large vacuum-sealable bag and cook in Sous Vide for 10 minutes at 162 F. Remove from the water bath and set aside.

Heat olive oil over medium heat in a large skillet. Add garlic and stir-fry for 1 minute. Stir in greens and season with salt. Sprinkle with fresh lemon juice and serve.

Brussel Sprouts in White Wine

Prep + Cook Time: 35 minutes | Servings: 4

Ingredients:

1 pound Brussels sprouts, trimmed

½ cup extra virgin olive oil

½ cup white wine

Salt and black pepper to taste

2 tbsp fresh parsley, finely chopped

2 garlic cloves, crushed

Directions:

Place Brussels sprouts in a large vacuum-sealable bag with three tablespoons of olive oil. Cook in Sous Vide for 15 minutes at 180 F. Remove from the bag.

In a large, non-stick grill pan, heat up the remaining olive oil. Add Brussels sprouts, crushed garlic, salt, and pepper. Briefly grill, shaking the pan a couple of times until lightly charred on all sides. Add wine and bring it to a boil. Stir well and remove from the heat. Top with finely chopped parsley and serve.

Beetroot & Goat Cheese Salad

Prep + Cook Time: 2 hours 20 minutes | Servings: 3

Ingredients:

1 lb beetroot, cut into wedges

½ cup almonds, blanched

2 tbsp hazelnuts, skinned

2 tsp olive oil

1 clove garlic, finely minced

1 tsp cumin powder

1 tsp lemon zest

Salt to taste

½ cup goat cheese, crumbled

Fresh mint leaves to garnish

Dressing:

2 tbsp olive oil

1 tbsp apple cider vinegar

Directions:

Make a water bath, place the Sous Vide in it, and set to 183 F.

Place the beetroots in a vacuum-sealable bag. Release air by the water displacement method, seal and submerge the bag in the water bath and set the timer for 2 hours. Once the timer has stopped, remove and unseal the bag. Place the beetroot aside.

Put a pan over medium heat, add almonds and hazelnuts, and toast for 3 minutes. Transfer to a cutting board and chop. Add oil to the same pan, place garlic and cumin. Cook for 30 seconds. Turn heat off. In a bowl, add the goat cheese, almond mixture, lemon zest, and garlic mixture. Mix. Whisk olive oil and vinegar and set aside. Serve as a side dish.

Cauliflower Broccoli Soup

Prep + Cook Time: 70 minutes | Servings: 2

Ingredients:

1 medium cauliflower, cut into small florets

½ lb broccoli, cut into small florets

1 green bell pepper, chopped

1 onion, diced

1 tsp olive oil

1 clove garlic, crushed

½ cup vegetable stock

½ cup skimmed milk

Directions:

Make a water bath, place the Sous Vide in it, and set it to 185 F.

Place the cauliflower, broccoli, bell pepper, and white onion in a vacuum-sealable bag and pour olive oil into it. Release air by the water displacement method and seal the bag. Submerge the bag in the water bath. Set the timer for 50 minutes and cook.

Once the timer has stopped, remove the bag and unseal. Transfer the vegetables to a blender, add garlic and milk, and puree to smooth.

Place a pan over medium heat, add the vegetable puree and vegetable stock and simmer for 3 minutes. Season with salt and pepper. Serve warm as a side dish.

Buttered Peas with Mint

Prep + Cook Time: 25 minutes | Servings: 2

Ingredients:

1 tbsp butter

½ cup snow peas

1 tbsp mint leaves, chopped

A pinch salt

Sugar to taste

Directions:

Make a water bath, place Sous Vide in it, and set to 183 F. Place all the ingredients in a vacuum-sealable bag. Release air by the water displacement method, seal and submerge in the bath. Cook for 15 minutes.

Once the timer has stopped, remove and unseal the bag. Transfer the ingredients to a serving plate. Serve as a condiment.

Brussels Sprouts in Sweet Syrup

Prep + Cook Time: 75 minutes | Servings: 3

Ingredients:

4 lb Brussels sprouts, halved

3 tbsp olive oil

¾ cup fish sauce

3 tbsp water

2 tbsp sugar

1 ½ tbsp rice vinegar

2 tsp lime juice

3 red chilies, sliced thinly

2 cloves garlic, minced

Directions:

Make a water bath, place Sous Vide in it, and set to 183 F. Pour Brussels sprouts, salt, and oil in a vacuum-sealable bag, release air by the water displacement method, seal and submerge the bag in the water bath. Set the timer for 50 minutes.

Once the timer has stopped, remove the bag, unseal, and transfer the Brussels sprouts to a foiled baking sheet. Preheat a broiler to high, place the baking sheet in it, and broil for 6 minutes. Pour the Brussels sprouts in a bowl.

Make the sauce: in a bowl, add the remaining listed cooking ingredients and stir. Add the sauce to the Brussels sprouts and toss evenly. Serve as a side dish.

Radish with Herb Cheese

Prep + Cook Time: 1 hour 15 minutes | Servings: 3

Ingredients:

10 oz goat cheese

4 oz cream cheese

¼ cup red bell pepper, minced

3 tbsp pesto

3 tsp lemon juice

2 tbsp parsley

2 clove garlic

9 large radishes, sliced.

Directions:

Make a water bath, place Sous Vide in it, and set to 181 F.Place the radish slices in a vacuum-sealable bag, release air and seal it. Submerge the bag in the water bath and set the timer for 1 hour.

In a bowl, mix the remaining listed ingredients and pour the mixture into a piping bag. Set aside. Once the timer has stopped, remove the bag and unseal. Arrange the radish slices on a serving platter and pipe the cheese mixture on each slice. Serve as a snack.

Balsamic Braised Cabbage

Prep + Cook Time: 1 hour 45 minutes | Servings: 3

Ingredients:

1 lb red cabbage, quartered and core removed

1 shallot, thinly sliced

2 cloves garlic, thinly sliced

½ tbsp balsamic vinegar

½ tbsp unsalted butter

Salt to taste

Directions:

Make a water bath, place Sous Vide in it, and set to 185 F. Divide cabbage and remaining ingredients into 2 vacuum-sealable bags. Release air by the water displacement method and seal the bags. Submerge them in the water bath and set the timer to cook for 1 hour 30 minutes.

Once the timer has stopped, remove and unseal the bags. Transfer the cabbage with juices into serving plates. Season with salt and vinegar to taste. Serve as a side dish.

Poached Tomatoes

Prep + Cook Time: 45 minutes | Servings: 3

Ingredients:

4 cups cherry tomatoes

5 tbsp olive oil

½ tbsp fresh rosemary leaves, minced

½ tbsp fresh thyme leaves, minced

Salt and black pepper to taste

Directions:

Make a water bath, place Sous Vide in it, and set to 131 F. Divide the listed ingredients into 2 vacuum-sealable bags, season with salt and pepper. Release air by the water displacement method and seal the bags. Submerge them in the water bath and set the timer to cook for 30 minutes.

Once the timer has stopped, remove the bags and unseal. Transfer the tomatoes with the juices into a bowl. Serve as a side dish.

Ratatouille

Prep + Cook Time: 2 hours 10 minutes | Servings: 3

Ingredients:

2 zucchinis, sliced

2 tomatoes, chopped

2 red capsicum, seeded and cut into 2-inch dices

1 small eggplant, sliced

1 onion, cut into 1-inch dices

Salt to taste

½ red pepper flakes

8 cloves garlic, crushed

2 ½ tbsp olive oil

5 sprigs + 2 sprigs Basil Leaves

Directions:

Make a water bath, place Sous Vide in it, and set to 185 F. Place the tomatoes, zucchini, onion, bell pepper and eggplant each in 5 separate vacuum-sealable bags. Put garlic, basil leaves, and 1 tablespoon of olive oil in each bag. Release air by the water displacement method, seal and submerge the bags in the water bath and set the timer for 20 minutes.

Once the timer has stopped, remove the bag with the tomatoes. Set aside. Reset the timer for 30 minutes. Once the timer has stopped, remove the bags with the zucchinis and red bell peppers. Set aside. Reset the timer for 1 hour.

Once the timer has stopped, remove the remaining bags and discard garlic and basil leaves. In a bowl, add tomatoes and use a spoon to mash them lightly. Chop the remaining vegetables and add to the tomatoes. Season with salt, red pepper flakes, remaining olive oil, and basil. Serve as a side dish.

Tomato Soup

Prep + Cook Time: 60 minutes | Servings: 3

Ingredients:

2 lb tomatoes, halved

1 onion, diced

1 celery stick, chopped

3 tbsp olive oil

1 tbsp tomato puree

A pinch sugar

1 bay leaf

Directions:

Make a water bath, place Sous Vide in it, and set to 185 F. Place all the listed ingredients except salt in bowl and toss. Put them in a vacuum-sealable bag. Release air by the water displacement method, seal and submerge the bag into the water bath. Set the timer for 40 minutes.

Once the timer has stopped, remove the bag and unseal. Puree the ingredients using a blender. Pour the blended tomato into a pot and set it over medium heat. Season with salt and cook for 10 minutes. Dish soup into bowls and cool. Serve warm with a side of low- carb bread.

Braised Beetroot

Prep + Cook Time: 1 hour 15 minutes | Servings: 3

Ingredients:

2 beets, peeled and sliced into 1 cm inches

⅓ cup balsamic vinegar

½ tsp olive oil

⅓ cup toasted walnuts

⅓ cup Grana Padano cheese, grated

Salt and black pepper to taste

Directions:

Make a water bath, place Sous Vide in it, and set to 183 F. Place the beets, vinegar, and salt in a vacuum-sealable bag. Release air by the water displacement method, seal and submerge the bag in the water bath. Set the timer for 1 hour.

Once the timer has stopped, remove and unseal the bag. Transfer the beets to a bowl, add olive oil and toss. Sprinkle walnuts and cheese over it. Serve as a side dish.

Eggplant Lasagna

Prep + Cook Time: 3 hours | Servings: 3

Ingredients:

1 lb eggplants, peeled and thinly sliced

1 tsp salt

1 cup tomato sauce, divided into 3

2 oz fresh mozzarella, thinly sliced

1 oz Parmesan cheese, grated

2 oz Italian blend cheese, grated

3 tbsp fresh basil, chopped

<u>Topping:</u>

½ tbsp macadamia nuts, toasted and chopped

1 oz Parmesan cheese, grated

1 oz italian blend cheese, grated

Directions:

Make a water bath, place Sous Vide in it, and set to 183 F. Season eggplants with salt. Lay a vacuum-sealable bag on its side, make a layer of half the eggplant, spread one portion of tomato sauce, layer mozzarella, then parmesan, then cheese blend, then basil. Top with the second portion of tomato sauce.

Seal the bag carefully by the water displacement method, keeping it flat as possible. Submerge the bag flat in the water bath. Set the timer for 2 hours and cook. Release air 2 to 3 times within the first 30 minutes as eggplant releases gas as it cooks.

Once the timer has stopped, remove the bag gently and poke one corner of the bag using a pin to release liquid from the bag. Lay the bag flat on a serving plate, cut open the top of it and gently slide the lasagna onto the plate. Top with remaining tomato sauce, macadamia nuts, cheese blend, and Parmesan cheese. Melt and brown the cheese using a torch.

Mushroom Soup

Prep + Cook Time: 50 minutes | Servings: 3

Ingredients:

1 lb mixed mushrooms

2 onions, diced

3 cloves garlic

2 sprigs parsley leaves, chopped

2 tbsp thyme powder

2 tbsp olive oil

2 cups cream

2 cups vegetable stock

Directions:

Make a water bath, place Sous Vide in it, and set to 185 F. Place the mushrooms, onion, and celery in a vacuum-sealable bag. Release air by the water displacement method, seal and submerge the bag in the water bath. Set the timer for 30 minutes. Once the timer has stopped, remove and unseal the bag.

Blend the ingredients from the bag in a blender. Put a pan over medium heat, add olive oil. Once it starts to heat, add in pureed mushrooms and the remaining ingredients, except for the cream. Cook for 10 minutes. Turn off heat and add cream. Stir well and serve.

Vegetarian Parmesan Risotto

Prep + Cook Time: 65 minutes | Servings: 5

Ingredients:

2 cups Arborio rice

½ cup plain white rice

1 cup veggie stock

1 cup water

6-8 ounces Parmesan cheese, grated

1 onion, chopped

1 tbsp butter

Salt and black pepper to taste

Directions:

Prepare a water bath and place Sous Vide in it. Set to 185 F. Melt the butter in a saucepan over medium heat. Add onions, rice and spices and cook for a few minutes. Transfer to a vacuum-sealable bag. Release air by the water displacement method, seal and submerge the bag in water bath. Set the timer for 50 minutes. Once the timer has stopped, remove the bag ans stir in the Parmesan cheese.

Green Soup

Prep + Cook Time: 55 minutes | Servings: 3

Ingredients:

4 cups vegetable stock

1 tbsp olive oil

1 clove garlic, crushed

1-inch ginger, sliced

1 tsp coriander powder

1 large zucchini, diced

3 cups kale

2 cups broccoli, cut into florets

1 Lime, juiced and zested

Directions:

Make a water bath, place Sous Vide in it, and set to 185 F. Place the broccoli, zucchini, kale, and parsley in a vacuum-sealable bag. Release air by the water displacement method, seal and submerge the bag in the water bath. Set the timer for 30 minutes.

Once the timer has stopped, remove and unseal the bag. Add the steamed ingredients to a blender with garlic and ginger. Puree to smooth. Pour the green puree into a pot and add the remaining listed ingredients. Put the pot over medium heat and simmer for 10 minutes. Serve as a light dish.

Mixed Vegetable Soup

Prep + Cook Time: 55 minutes | Servings: 3

Ingredients:

1 sweet onion, sliced

1 tsp garlic powder

2 cups zucchini, cut in small dices

3 oz Parmesan rind

2 cups baby spinach

2 tbsp olive oil

1 tsp red pepper flakes

2 cups vegetable stock

1 sprig rosemary

Salt to taste

Directions:

Make a water bath, place Sous Vide in it, and set to 185 F. Toss all the ingredients with olive oil except the garlic and salt, and place them in a vacuum-sealable bag. Release air by water displacement method, seal and submerge the bag in the water bath. Set the timer for 30 minutes.

Once the timer has stopped, remove and unseal the bag. Discard the rosemary. Pour the remaining ingredients into a pot and add salt and garlic powder. Put the pot over medium heat and simmer for 10 minutes. Serve as a light dish.

Smoked Paprika Veggie Wontons

Prep + Cook Time: 5 hours 15 minutes | Servings: 9)

Ingredients:

10 ounces wonton wraps

10 ounces veggies by choice, grated

2 eggs

1 tsp olive oil

½ tsp chili powder

½ tsp smoked paprika

½ tsp garlic powder

Salt and black pepper to taste

Directions:

Prepare a water bath and place the Sous Vide in it. Set to 165 F.

Beat the eggs along with the spices. Stir in the veggies and oil. Pour the mixture into a vacuum-sealable bag-Release air by the water displacement method, seal and submerge the bag in water bath.Set the timer for 5 hours.

Once the timer has stopped, remove the bag and transfer to a bowl. Divide the mixture between the ravioli, wrap and pinch the edges to seal. Cook in a boiling water for 4 minutes over medium heat.

Quinoa & Celeriac Miso Dish

Prep + Cook Time: 2 hours 25 minutes | Servings: 6

Ingredients

1 celeriac, chopped

1 tbsp miso paste

6 cloves garlic

5 sprigs thyme

1 tsp onion powder

3 tbsp ricotta cheese

1 tbsp mustard seeds

Juice of ¼ a large lemon

5 cherry tomatoes roughly cut

Chopped parsley

8 ounces vegan butter

8 ounce cooked quinoa

Directions

Prepare a water bath and place the Sous Vide in it. Set to 186 F.

Meanwhile, heat a skillet over medium heat and add the garlic, thyme, mustard seeds. Cook for about 2 minutes. Add butter and stirring until browned. Combine with onion powder and set aside.

Allow to cool at room temperature. Place the celeriac in a vacuum-sealable bag. Release air by the water displacement method, seal and submerge the bag in the water bath. Cook for 2 hours.

Once the timer has stopped, remove the bag and transfer to a skillet and stirring until golden brown. Season with miso. Set aside. Heat a pan over medium heat, add tomatoes, mustard and quinoa. Combine with lemon juice and parsley. Serve by mixing the celeriac and tomato mix.

Radish & Basil Salad

Prep + Cook Time: 50 minutes | Servings: 2

Ingredients:

20 small radishes, trimmed

1 tbsp white wine vinegar

¼ cup chopped basil

½ cup feta cheese

1 tsp sugar

1 tbsp water

¼ tsp salt

Directions:

Prepare a water bath and place the Sous Vide in it. Set to 200 F. Place the radishes in a large vacuum-sealable bag and add vinegar, sugar, salt and water. Shake to combine. Release air by the water displacement method, seal and submerge in water bath. Cook for 30 minutes. Once the timer has stopped, remove the bag and let cool in an ice bath. Serve warm. Serve tossed with the basil and feta.

Bell Pepper Mix

Prep + Cook Time: 35 minutes | Servings: 2

Ingredients:

1 red bell pepper, chopped

1 yellow bell pepper, chopped

1 green bell pepper, chopped

1 large orange bell pepper, chopped

Salt to taste

Directions:

Make a water bath, place Sous Vide in it, and set to 183 F. Place all the bell peppers with salt in a vacuum-sealable bag. Release air by the water displacement method, seal and submerge in the water bath. Set the timer for 15 minutes. Once the timer has stopped, remove and unseal the bag. Serve bell peppers with its juices as a side dish.

Cilantro Turmeric Quinoa

Prep + Cook Time: 105 minutes | Servings: 6

Ingredients:

3 cups quinoa

2 cups heavy cream

½ cup water

3 tbsp cilantro leaves

2 tsp turmeric powder

1 tbsp butter

½ tbsp salt

Directions:

Prepare a water bath and place the Sous Vide in it. Set to 180 F.

Place all the ingredients in a vacuum-sealable bag. Stir to combine well. Release air by the water displacement method, seal and submerge the bag in water bath. Set the timer for 90 minutes. Once the timer has stopped, remove the bag. Serve warm.

Oregano White Bean s

Prep + Cook Time: 5 hours 15 minutes | Servings: 8

Ingredients:

12 ounces white beans

1 cup tomato paste

8 ounces veggie stock

1 tbsp sugar

3 tbsp butter

1 cup chopped onions

1 bell pepper, chopped

1 tbsp oregano

2 tsp paprika

Directions:

Prepare a water bath and place the Sous Vide in it. Set to 185 F.

Combine all the ingredients in a vacuum-sealable bag. Stir to combine. Release air by the water displacement method, seal and submerge the bag in water bath.Set the timer for 5 hours. Once the timer has stopped, remove the bag. Serve warm.

Potato & Date Salad

Prep + Cook Time: 3 hours 15 minutes | Servings: 6

Ingredients:

2 pounds potatoes, cubed

5 ounces dates, chopped

½ cup crumbled goat cheese

1 tsp oregano

1 tbsp olive oil

1 tbsp lemon juice

3 tbsp butter

1 tsp cilantro

1 tsp salt

1 tbsp chopped parsley

¼ tsp garlic powder

Directions:

Prepare a water bath and place the Sous Vide in it. Set to 190 F.

Place the potatoes, butter, dates, oregano, cilantro, and salt in a vacuum-sealable bag. Release air by the water displacement method, seal and submerge the bag in water bath. Set the timer for 3 hours.

Once the timer has stopped, remove the bag and transfer to a bowl. Whisk together the olive oil, lemon juice, parsley, and garlic powder and drizzle over the salad. If using cheese, sprinkle it over.

Paprika Grits

Prep + Cook Time: 3 hours 10 minutes | Servings: 4

Ingredients:

10 ounces grits

4 tbsp butter

1 ½ tsp paprika

10 ounces water

½ tsp garlic salt

Directions:

Prepare a water bath and place the Sous Vide in it. Set to 180 F.

Place all the ingredients in a vacuum-sealable bag. Stir with spoon to combine well. Release air by the water displacement method, seal and submerge the bag in water bath.Set the timer for 3 hours. Once the timer has stopped, remove the bag. Divide between 4 serving bowls.

Grape Vegetable Mix

Prep + Cook Time 105 minutes | Servings: 9)

Ingredients:

8 sweet potatoes, sliced

2 red onions, sliced

4 ounces tomato, pureed

1 tsp minced garlic

Salt and black pepper to taste

1 tsp grape juice

Directions:

Prepare a water bath and place Sous Vide in it. Set to 183 F. Place all the ingredients with ¼ cup water in a vacuum-sealable bag.Release air by the water displacement method, seal and submerge the bag in water bath. Set the timer for 90 minutes. Once the timer has stopped, remove the bag. Serve warm.

Minty Chickpea and Mushroom Bowl

Prep + Cook Time: 4 hours 15 minutes | Servings: 8

Ingredients:

9 ounces mushrooms

3 cups veggie broth

1 pound chickpeas, soaked overnight and drained

1 tsp butter

1 tsp paprika

1 tbsp mustard

2 tbsp tomato juice

1 tsp salt

¼ cup chopped mint

1 tbsp olive oil

Directions:

Prepare a water bath and place the Sous Vide in it. Set to 195 F. Place broth and chickpeas in a vacuum-sealable bag. Release air by the water displacement method, seal and submerge the bag in water bath.Set the timer for 4 hours.

Once the timer has stopped, remove the bag. Heat oil in a pan over medium heat. Add in mushrooms, tomato juice, paprika, salt, and mustard. Cook for 4 minutes. Drain the chickpeas and add them to the pan. Cook for another 4 minutes. Stir in butter and mint.

Vegetable Caponata

Prep + Cook Time: 2 hours 15 minutes | Servings: 4

Ingredients:

4 canned plum tomatoes, crushed

2 bell peppers, sliced

2 zucchinis, sliced

½ onion, sliced

2 eggplants, sliced

6 garlic cloves, minced

2 tbsp olive oil

6 basil leaves

Salt and black pepper to taste

Directions:

Prepare a water bath and place the Sous Vide in it. Set to 185 F. Combine all of the ingredients in a vacuum-sealable bag. Release air by the water displacement method, seal and submerge the bag in water bath.Set the timer for 2 hours. Once the timer has stopped, transfer to a serving platter.

Braised Swiss Chard with Lime

Prep + Cook Time: 25 minutes | Servings: 2

2 pounds Swiss chard

4 tbsp of extra virgin olive oil

2 garlic cloves, crushed

1 whole lime, juiced

2 tsps sea salt

Directions:

Thoroughly rinse Swiss chard and drain in a colander. Using a sharp paring knife roughly chop and transfer to a large bowl. Stir in 4 tablespoons of olive oil, crushed garlic, lime juice, and sea salt. Transfer to a large vacuum-sealable bag and seal. Cook en sous vide for 10 minutes at 180 F.

Root Veggie Mash

Prep + Cook Time: 3 hours 15 minutes | Servings: 4

Ingredients:

2 parsnips, peeled and chopped

1 turnip, peeled and chopped

1 large sweet potatoes, peeled and chopped

1 tbsp butter

Salt and black pepper to taste

Pinch of nutmeg

¼ tsp thyme

Directions:

Prepare a water bath and place Sous Vide in it. Set to 185 F. Place the veggies in a vacuum-sealable bag. Release air by the water displacement method, seal and submerge in water bath.Cook for 3 hours. Once done, remove the bag and mash the veggies with a potato masher. Stir in the remaining ingredients.

Cabbage & Pepper in Tomato Sauce

Prep + Cook Time: 4 hours 45 minutes | Servings: 6

Ingredients:

2 pounds cabbage, sliced

1 cup sliced bell pepper

1 cup tomato paste

2 onions, sliced

1 tbsp sugar

Salt and black pepper to taste

1 tbsp cilantro

1 tbsp olive oil

Directions:

Prepare a water bath and place the Sous Vide in it. Set to 184 F.

Place the cabbage and onion in a vacuum-sealable bag and season with the spices. Add in tomato paste and stir to combine well. Release air by the water displacement method, seal and submerge the bag in water bath.Set the timer for 4 hours and 30 minutes. Once the timer has stopped, remove the bag.

Mustardy Lentil & Tomato Dish

Prep + Cook Time: 105 minutes | Servings: 8

Ingredients:

2 cups lentils

1 can chopped tomatoes, undrained

1 cup green peas

3 cups veggie stock

3 cups water

1 onion, chopped

1 carrot, sliced

1 tbsp butter

2 tbsp mustard

1 tsp red pepper flakes

2 tbsp lime juice

Salt and black pepper to taste

Directions:

Prepare a water bath and place Sous Vide in it. Set to 192 F. Place all the ingredients in a large vacuum-sealable bag. Release air by water displacement method, seal and submerge in bath. Cook for 90 minutes. Once the timer has stopped, remove the bag and transfer to a large bowl and stir before serving.

Bell Pepper Rice Pilaf with Raisins

Prep + Cook Time: 3 hours 10 minutes | Servings: 6

Ingredients:

2 cups white rice

2 cups veggie stock

⅔ cup water

3 tbsp raisins, chopped

2 tbsp sour cream

½ cup chopped red onion

1 bell pepper, chopped

Salt and black pepper to taste

1 tsp thyme

Directions:

Prepare a water bath and place the Sous Vide in it. Set to 180 F.

Place all the ingredients in a vacuum-sealable bag. Stir to combine well. Release air by the water displacement method, seal and submerge the bag in water bath.Set the timer for 3 hours. Once the timer has stopped, remove the bag. Serve warm.

Yogurt Caraway Soup

Prep + Cook Time: 2 hours 20 minutes | Servings: 4

Ingredients

1 tbsp olive oil

1½ tsp caraway seeds

1 medium onion, diced

1 leek, halved and thinly sliced

Salt to taste

2 pounds carrots, chopped

1 bay leaf

3 cups vegetable broth

½ cup whole milk yogurt

Apple cider vinegar

Fresh dill fronds

Directions

Prepare a water bath and place the Sous Vide in it. Set to 186 F. Heat olive oil in a large skillet over medium heat and add caraway seeds. Toast them for 1 minute. Add in onion, salt and leek, Sauté for 5-7 minutes or until tender. Combine the onion, bay leaf, carrots and 1/2 tbsp of salt into a large bowl.

Distribute the mixture in a vacuum-sealable bag. Release air by the water displacement method, seal and submerge the bag in the water bath. Cook for 2 hours.

Once the timer has stopped, remove the bag and pour into a bowl. Add in vegetable broth and blend. Stir in yogurt. Season the soup with some salt and vinegar and serve garnished dill fronds.

Buttery Summer Squash

Prep + Cook Time: 1 hour 35 minutes | Servings: 4

Ingredients

2 tbsp butter

¾ cup onion, chopped

1½ pounds summer squash, sliced

Salt and black pepper to taste

½ cup whole milk

2 large whole eggs

½ cup crumbled plain potato chips

Directions

Prepare a water bath and place the Sous Vide in it. Set to 175 F

Meanwhile, grease a few jars. Heat a large skillet over medium heat and melt the butter. Add in onions and sauté for 7 minutes. Add the squash, season with salt and pepper and sauté for 10 minutes. Divide the mix in the jars. Allow it cool and set aside.

Whisk the milk, salt and eggs in a bowl. Season with pepper. Pour the mixture over the jars, seal and submerge the jars in the water bath. Cook for 60 minutes. Once the timer has stopped, remove the jars and allow cooling for 5 minutes. Serve over potato chips.

Curry Ginger & Nectarine Chutney

Prep + Cook Time: 60 minutes | Servings: 3

Ingredients

½ cup granulated sugar

½ cup water

¼ cup white wine vinegar

1 garlic clove, minced

¼ cup white onion, finely chopped

Juice of 1 lime

2 tsp grated fresh ginger

2 tsp curry powder

A pinch of red pepper flakes

Salt and black pepper to taste

Pepper flakes to taste

4 large pieces nectarine, sliced into wedges

¼ cup chopped up fresh basil

Directions

Prepare a water bath and place the Sous Vide in it. Set to 168 F.

Heat a saucepan over medium heat and combine the water, sugar, white wine vinegar, and garlic. Moving until the sugar soften. Add lime juice, onion, curry powder, ginger, and red pepper flakes. Season with salt and black pepper. Stir well. Place the mixture in a vacuum-sealable bag. Release air by the water displacement method, seal and submerge the bag in the water bath. Cook for 40 minutes.

Once the timer has stopped, remove the bag and place in ice bath. Transfer the food on a serving plate. Garnish with basil.

Rosemary Russet Potatoes Confit

Prep + Cook Time: 1 hour 15 minutes | Servings: 4

Ingredients

1 pound brown russet potatoes, chopped

Salt to taste

¼ tsp ground white pepper

1 tsp chopped fresh rosemary

2 tbsp whole butter

1 tbsp corn oil

Directions

Prepare a water bath and place Sous Vide in it. Set to 192 F. Season potatoes with rosemary, salt and pepper. Combine the potatoes with butter and oil. Place in a vacuum-sealable bag. Release air by the water displacement method, seal and submerge the bag in the water bath. Cook for 60 minutes. Once the timer has stopped, remove the bag and transfer into a large bowl. Garnish with butter and serve.

Curry Pears & Coconut Cream

Prep + Cook Time: 1 hour 10 minutes | Servings: 4

Ingredients

2 pears, cored, peeled and sliced

1 tbsp curry powder

2 tbsp coconut cream

Directions

Prepare a water bath and place the Sous Vide in it. Set to 186 F.

Combine all the ingredients and place in a vacuum-sealable bag. Release air by the water displacement method, seal and submerge the bag in the water bath. Cook for 60 minutes. Once the timer has stopped, remove the bag and transfer to a large bowl. Divide in serving plates and serve.

Soft Broccoli Purée

Prep + Cook Time: 2 hours 15 minutes | Servings: 4

Ingredients

1 head broccoli, cut into florets

½ tsp garlic powder

Salt to taste

1 tbsp butter

1 tbsp heavy whipping cream

Directions

Prepare a water bath and place the Sous Vide in it. Set to 183 F. Combine the broccoli, salt, garlic powder, and heavy cream. Place in a vacuum-sealable bag. Release air by the water displacement method, seal and submerge the bag in the water bath. Cook for 2 hours.

Once the timer has stopped, remove the bag and transfer into a blender to pulse. Season and serve.

Delicious Chutney of Dates & Mangoes

Prep + Cook Time: 1 hour 45 minutes | Servings: 4

Ingredients

2 pounds mangoes, chopped

1 small onion, diced

½ cup light brown sugar

¼ cup dates

2 tbsp apple cider vinegar

2 tbsp freshly squeezed lemon juice

1½ tsp yellow mustard seeds

1½ tsp coriander seeds

Salt to taste

¼ tsp curry powder

¼ tsp dried turmeric

⅛ tsp cayenne

Directions

Prepare a water bath and place the Sous Vide in it. Set to 183 F.

Combine all the ingredients. Place in a vacuum-sealable bag. Release air by the water displacement method, seal and submerge the bag in the water bath. Cook for 90 minutes. Once the timer has stopped, remove the bag and pour into a pot.

Mandarin & Green Bean Salad with Walnuts

Prep + Cook Time: 1 hour 10 minutes | Servings: 8)

Ingredients

2 pounds green beans, trimmed

2 mandarins

2 tbsp butter

Salt to taste

2 oz walnuts

Directions

Prepare a water bath and place the Sous Vide in it. Set to 186 F. Combine the green beans, salt and butter. Place in a vacuum-sealable bag. Add in mandarin zest and juice. Release air by the water displacement method, seal and submerge the bag in the water bath. Cook for 1 hour. Once the timer has stopped, remove the bag and transfer to a serving platter. Top with mandarin zest and walnuts.

Green Pea Cream with Nutmeg

Prep + Cook Time: 1 hour 10 minutes | Servings: 8)

Ingredients

1 pound fresh green peas

1 cup whipping cream

¼ cup butter

1 tbsp cornstarch

¼ tsp ground nutmeg

4 cloves

2 bay leaves

Black pepper to taste

Directions

Prepare a water bath and place the Sous Vide in it. Set to 184 F. Combine the cornstarch, nutmeg and cream into a bowl. Whisk until the cornstarch soften.

Place the mixture in a vacuum-sealable bag. Release air by the water displacement method, seal and submerge the bag in the water bath. Cook for 1 hour. Once the timer has stopped, extract the bag and remove the bay leaf. Serve.

Easy Broccoli Puree

Prep + Cook Time: 60 minutes | Servings: 4

Ingredients

1 head broccoli

1 cup vegetable stock

3 tbsp butter

Salt to taste

Directions

Prepare a water bath and place the Sous Vide in it. Set to 186 F.

Combine the broccoli, butter and vegetable stock. Place in a vacuum-sealable bag. Release air by the water displacement method, seal and submerge the bag in the water bath. Cook for 45 minutes.

Once the timer has stopped, remove the bag and drain. Reserve the cooking juices. Put the broccoli into a blender and puree until smooth. Pour some cooking juices. Season with salt and pepper to serve.

Red Chili Broccoli Soup

Prep + Cook Time: 1 hour 25 minutes | Servings: 8)

Ingredients

2 tbsp olive oil

1 large onion, diced

2 garlic cloves, sliced

Salt to taste

⅛ tsp crushed red chili flakes

1 broccoli head, cut into florets

1 apple, peeled and diced

6 cups vegetable broth

Directions

Prepare a water bath and place the Sous Vide in it. Set to 183 F.

Heat a skillet over medium heat with the oil, until shimmer. Sauté the onion, 1/4 tbsp of salt and garlic for 7 minutes. Add in chili flakes and mix well. Remove from the heat. Allow cooling.

Place the apple, broccoli, onion mix and 1/4 tbsp of salt in a vacuum-sealable bag. Release air by the water displacement method, seal and submerge the bag in the water bath. Cook for 1 hour.

Once the timer has stopped, remove the bag and transfer to a pot. Pour in vegetable broth and blend. Season with salt and serve.

Allspice Miso Corn with Sesame & Honey

Prep + Cook Time: 45 minutes | Servings: 4

Ingredients

4 ears of corn

6 tbsp butter

3 tbsp red miso paste

1 tsp honey

1 tsp allspice

1 tbsp canola oil

1 scallion, thinly sliced

1 tsp toasted sesame seeds

Directions

Prepare a water bath and place the Sous Vide in it. Set to 183 F. Clean the corn and cut the ears. Cover each corn with 2 tbsp of butter. Place in a vacuum-sealable bag. Release air by the water displacement method, seal and submerge the bag in the water bath. Cook for 30 minutes.

Meanwhile, combine 4 tbsp of butter, 2 tbsp of miso paste, honey, canola oil, and allspice in a bowl. Stir well. Set aside. Once the timer has stopped, remove the bag and sear the corn. Spread the miso mixture on top. Garnish with sesame oil and scallions.

Creamy Gnocchi with Peas

Prep + Cook Time: 1 hour 50 minutes | Servings: 2

Ingredients

1 pack gnocchi

1 tbsp butter

½ thinly sliced sweet onion

Salt and black pepper to taste

½ cup frozen peas

¼ cup heavy cream

½ cup grated Pecorino Romano cheese

Directions

Prepare a water bath and place the Sous Vide in it. Set to 183 F. Place the gnocchi in a vacuum-sealable bag. Release air by the water displacement method, seal and submerge the bag in the water bath. Cook for 1 hour and 30 minutes.

Once the timer has stopped, remove the bag and set aside. Heat a skillet over medium heat with butter and sauté the onion for 3 minutes. Add the frozen peas and cream and cook. Combine the gnocchi with the cream sauce, season with pepper and salt and serve in a plate.

Honey Apple & Arugula Salad

Prep + Cook Time: 3 hours 50 minutes | Servings: 4

Ingredients

2 tbsp honey

2 apples, cored, halved and sliced

½ cup walnuts, toasted and chopped

½ cup shaved Grana Padano cheese

4 cups arugula

Sea salt to taste

Dressing

¼ cup olive oil

1 tbsp white wine vinegar

1 tsp Dijon mustard

1 garlic clove, minced

Salt to taste

Directions

Prepare a water bath and place the Sous Vide in it. Set to 158 F. Place the honey in a glass bowl and heat for 30 seconds, add the apples and mix well. Place it in a vacuum-sealable bag. Release air by the water displacement method, seal and submerge the bag in the water bath. Cook for 30 minutes.

Once the timer has stopped, remove the bag and transfer into an ice-water bath for 5 minutes. Refrigerate for 3 hours. Combine all the dressing ingredients in a jar and shake well. Allow cooling in the fridge for a moment.

In a bowl, mix the arugula, walnuts, and Grana Padano cheese. Add the peach slices. Top with the dressing. Season with salt and pepper and serve.

Crabmeat with Lime Butter Sauce

Prep + Cook Time: 70 minutes | Servings: 4

Ingredients

6 garlic cloves, minced

Zest and juice from ½ lime

1 pound crabmeat

4 tbsp butter

Directions

Prepare a water bath and place the Sous Vide in it. Set to 137 F. Combine well the half of garlic, lime zest and half of lime juice. Set aside. Place the crabmeat, butter and lime mixture in a vacuum-sealable bag. Release air by the water displacement method, seal and submerge the bag in the water bath. Cook for 50 minutes. Once the timer has stopped, remove the bag. Discard the cooking juices.

Heat a saucepan over medium-low heat and pour in remaining butter, remaining lime mixture and remaining lime juice. Serve the crab in 4 ramekins, sprinkled with lime butter.

Speedy North-Style Salmon

Prep + Cook Time: 30 minutes | Servings: 4

Ingredients

1 tbsp olive oil

4 salmon fillets, skin-on

Salt and black pepper to taste

Zest and juice of 1 lemon

2 tbsp yellow mustard

2 tsp sesame oil

Directions

Prepare a water bath and place Sous Vide in it. Set to 114 F. Season salmon with salt and pepper. Combine lemon zest and juice, oil, and mustard. Place the salmon in 2 vacuum-sealable bags with the mustard mixture. Release air by the water displacement method, seal and submerge the bags in the bath. Cook for 20 minutes. Heat sesame oil in a skillet. Once the timer has stopped, remove the salmon and pat dry. Transfer the salmon into the skillet and sear for 30 seconds per side.

Tasty Trout with Mustard & Tamari Sauce

Prep + Cook Time: 35 minutes | Servings: 4

Ingredients

¼ cup olive oil

4 trout fillets, skinned and sliced

½ cup Tamari sauce

¼ cup light brown sugar

2 garlic cloves, minced

1 tbsp Coleman's mustard

Directions

Prepare a water bath and place Sous Vide in it. Set to 130 F. Combine the Tamari sauce, brown sugar, olive oil, and garlic. Place the trout in a vacuum-sealable bag with tamari mixture. Release air by the water displacement method, seal and submerge the bag in the water bath. Cook for 30 minutes.

Once the timer has stopped, remove the trout and pat dry with kitchen towel. Discard the cooking juices. Garnish with tamari sauce and mustard to serve.

Sesame Tuna with Ginger Sauce

Prep + Cook Time: 45 minutes | Servings: 6

Ingredients:

Tuna:

3 tuna steaks

Salt and black pepper to taste

⅓ cup olive oil

2 tbsp canola oil

½ cup black sesame seeds

½ cup white sesame seeds

Ginger Sauce:

1 inch ginger, grated

2 shallots, minced

1 red chili, minced

3 tbsp water

2 ½ lime juice

1 ½ tbsp rice vinegar

2 ½ tbsp soy sauce

1 tbsp fish sauce

1 ½ tbsp sugar

1 bunch green lettuce leaves

Directions:

Start with the sauce: place a small pan over low heat and add olive oil. Once it has heated, add ginger and chili. Cook for 3 minutes Add sugar and vinegar, stir and cook until sugar dissolves. Add water and bring to a boil. Add in soy sauce, fish sauce, and lime juice and cook for 2 minutes. Set aside to cool.

Make a water bath, place Sous Vide in it, and set to 110 F. Season the tuna with salt and pepper and place in 3 separate vacuum-sealable bag. Add olive oil, release air from the bag by the water displacement method, seal and submerge the bag in the water bath. Set the timer for 30 minutes.

Once the timer has stopped, remove and unseal the bag. Place tuna aside. Place a skillet over low heat and add canola oil. While heating, mix sesame seeds in a bowl. Pat dry tuna, coat them in sesame seeds and sear top and bottom in heated oil until seeds start to toast.

Slice tuna into thin strips. Layer a serving platter with lettuce and arrange tuna on the bed of lettuce. Serve with ginger sauce as a starter.

Divine Garlic-Lemon Crab Rolls

Prep + Cook Time: 60 minutes | Servings: 4

Ingredients

4 tbsp butter

1 pound cooked crabmeat

2 garlic cloves, minced

Zest and juice of ½ lemon

½ cup mayonnaise

1 fennel bulb, chopped

Salt and black pepper to taste

4 rolls, split, oiled, and toasted

Directions

Prepare a water bath and place Sous Vide in it. Set to 137 F. Combine garlic, lemon zest and 1/4 cup of lemon juice. Place the crabmeat in a vacuum-sealable bag with butter and lemon mix. Release air by the water displacement method, seal and submerge the bag in the water bath. Cook for 50 minutes.

Once the timer has stopped, remove the bag and transfer into a bowl. Discard the cooking juices. Combine the crabmeat with the remaining lemon juice, mayonnaise, fennel, dill, salt, and pepper. Fill the rolls with the crabmeat mixture before serving.

Spiced Charred Octopus with Lemon Sauce

Prep + Cook Time: 4 hours 15 minutes | Servings: 4

Ingredients

5 tbsp olive oil

1 pound octopus tentacles

Salt and black pepper to taste

2 tbsp lemon juice

1 tbsp lemon zest

1 tbsp minced fresh parsley

1 tsp thyme

1 tbsp paprika

Directions

Prepare a water bath and place the Sous Vide in it. Set to 179 F. Cut the tentacles into medium-size lengths. Season with salt and pepper. Place the lengths with olive oil in a vacuum-sealable bag. Release air by the water displacement method, seal and submerge the bag in the water bath. Cook for 4 hours.

Once the timer has stopped, remove the octopus and pat pat dry with kitchen towel. Discard the cooking juices. Sprinkle with olive oil.

Heat a grill over medium heat and sear the tentacles for 10-15 seconds per side. Set aside. Combine well the lemon juice, lemon zest, paprika, thyme and parsley. Top the octopus with lemon dressing.

Creole Prawn Kabobs

Prep + Cook Time: 50 minutes | Servings: 4

Ingredients

Zest and juice of 1 lemon

6 tbsp butter

2 garlic cloves, minced

Salt and white pepper to taste

1 tbsp Creole seasoning

1½ pounds prawns, deveined

1 tbsp minced fresh dill + for garnish

Lemon wedges

Directions

Prepare a water bath and place the Sous Vide in it. Set to 137 F.

Melt butter in a saucepan over medium heat and add in garlic, Creole seasoning, lemon zest and juice, salt and pepper. Cook for 5 minutes until the butter melted. Set aside and allow to cool.

Place the prawns in a vacuum-sealable bag with the butter mix. Release air by the water displacement method, seal and submerge the bag in the water bath. Cook for 30 minutes.

Once the timer has stopped, remove the prawns and pat dry with kitchen towel. Discard the cooking juices. Thread the prawns onto the kabobs and garnish with dill and squeeze lemon to serve.

Shrimp with Spicy Sauce

Prep + Cook Time: 40 minutes + Cooling Time | Servings: 5

Ingredients

2 pounds shrimp, deveined and peeled

1 cup tomato puree

2 tbsp horseradish sauce

1 tsp lemon juice

1 tsp Tabasco sauce

Salt and black pepper to taste

Directions

Prepare a water bath and place Sous Vide in it. Set to 137 F. Place shrimp in a vacuum-sealable bag. Release air by the water displacement method, seal and submerge bag in the bath. Cook for 30 minutes.

Once the timer has stopped, remove the bag and transfer into an ice water bath for 10 minutes. Allow to chill in the fridge for 1-6 hours. Combine well the tomato puree, horseradish sauce, soy sauce, lemon juice, Tabasco sauce, salt and pepper. Serve shrimp with the sauce.

Halibut with Shallots & Tarragon

Prep + Cook Time: 50 minutes | Servings: 2

Ingredients:

2 lb halibut filets

3 sprigs tarragon leaves

1 tsp garlic powder

1 tsp onion powder

Salt and white pepper to taste

2 ½ tsp + 2 tsp butter

2 shallots, peeled and halved

2 sprigs thyme

Lemon wedges for garnishing

Directions:

Make a water bath, place Sous Vide in it, and set to 124 F. Cut halibut filets into 3 piccccs cach and rub with salt, garlic powder, onion powder, and pepper. Place the filets, tarragon, and 2 ½ teaspoons of butter into 3 different vacuum-sealable bags. Release air by the water displacement method and seal the bags. Place them in the water bath and cook for 40 minutes.

Once the timer has stopped, remove and unseal the bags. Place a skillet over low heat and add the remaining butter. Once it is heated, remove the skin of the halibuts and pat dry. Add halibuts with shallots and thyme and sear bottom and top until crispy. Garnish with lemon wedges. Serve with a side of steamed vegetables.

Herb Butter Lemon Cod

Prep + Cook Time: 37 minutes | Servings: 6

Ingredients

8 tbsp butter

6 cod fillets

Salt and black pepper to taste

Zest of ½ lemon

1 tbsp minced fresh dill

½ tbsp minced fresh chives

½ tbsp minced fresh basil

½ tbsp minced fresh sage

Directions

Prepare a water bath and place the Sous Vide in it. Set to 134 F. Season the cod with salt and pepper. Place the cod and lemon zest in a vacuum-sealable bag.

In a separate vacuum-sealable bag, place the butter, half of dill, chives, basil, and sage. Release air by the water displacement method, seal and submerge both bags in the water bath. Cook for 30 minutes.

Once the timer has stopped, remove the cod and pat dry with kitchen towel. Discard the cooking juices. Remove the butter from the other bag and pour over the cod. Garnish with the remaining dill.

Grouper with Beurre Nantais

Prep + Cook Time: 45 minutes | Servings: 6

Ingredients:

<u>Grouper:</u>

2 lb grouper, cut into 3 pieces each

1 tsp cumin powder

½ tsp garlic powder

½ tsp onion powder

½ tsp coriander powder

¼ cup fish seasoning

¼ cup pecan oil

Salt and white pepper to taste

<u>Beurre Blanc:</u>

1 lb butter

2 tbsp apple cider vinegar

2 shallots, minced

1 tsp peppercorns, crushed

5 oz heavy cream,

Salt to taste

2 sprigs dill

1 tbsp lemon juice

1 tbsp saffron powder

Directions:

Make a water bath, place Sous Vide in it, and set to 132 F. Season the grouper pieces with salt and white pepper. Place in a vacuum-sealable bag, release air by the water displacement method, seal and submerge the bag in the water bath. Set the timer for 30 minutes. Mix the cumin, garlic, onion, coriander, and fish seasoning. Set aside.

Meanwhile, make the beurre blanc. Place a pan over medium heat and add, shallots, vinegar, and peppercorns. Cook to attain a syrup. Reduce heat to low and add butter, whisking continuously. Add dill, lemon juice, and saffron powder, stir continuously and cook for 2 minutes. Add cream and season with salt. Cook for 1 minute. Turn heat off and set aside.

Once the timer has stopped, remove and unseal the bag. Set a skillet over medium heat, add pecan oil. Pat dry the grouper and seasoning with the spice mixture and sear them in the heated oil. Serve grouper and beurre nantais with a side of steamed spinach.

Tuna Flakes

Prep + Cook Time: 1 hour 45 minutes | Servings: 4

Ingredients:

¼ lb tuna steak

1 tsp rosemary leaves

1 tsp thyme leaves

2 cups olive oil

1 clove garlic, minced

Directions:

Make a water bath, place Sous Vide in it, and set to 135 F. Place the tuna steak, salt, rosemary, garlic, thyme, and two tablespoons of oil in the vacuum-sealable bag. Release air by the water displacement method, seal and submerge the bag in the water bath. Set the timer for 1 hour 30 minutes.

Once the timer has stopped, remove the bag. Place the tuna in a bowl and set aside. Place a skillet over high heat, add the remaining olive oil. Once it has heated, pour over the tuna. Flake the tuna using two forks. Transfer and store in an airtight container with olive oil for up to a week. Serve in salads.

Buttered Scallops

Prep + Cook Time: 55 minutes | Servings: 3

Ingredients:

½ lb scallops

3 tsp butter (2 tsp for cooking + 1 tsp for searing)

Salt and black pepper to taste

Directions:

Make a water bath, place Sous Vide in it, and set to 140 F. Pat dry scallops using a paper towel. Place scallops, salt, 2 tablespoons of butter, and pepper in a vacuum-sealable bag. Release air by the water displacement method, seal and submerge the bag in the water bath and set the timer for 40 minutes.

Once the timer has stopped, remove and unseal the bag. Pat dry the scallops using a paper towel and set aside. Set a skillet over medium heat and the remaining butter. Once it has melted, sear the scallops on both sides until golden brown. Serve with a side of buttered mixed vegetables.

Minty Sardines

Prep + Cook Time: 1 hour 20 minutes | Servings: 3

Ingredients:

2 pounds sardines

¼ cup olive oil

3 garlic cloves, crushed

1 large lemon, freshly juiced

2 sprigs fresh mint

Salt and black pepper to taste

Directions:

Wash and clean each fish but keep the skin. Pat dry using a kitchen paper.

In a large bowl, combine olive oil with garlic, lemon juice, fresh mint, salt, and pepper. Place the sardines in a large vacuum-sealable bag along with the marinade. Cook in a water bath for one hour at 104 F. Remove from the bath and drain but reserve the sauce. Drizzle fish with sauce and steamed leek.

Sea Bream in White Wine

Prep + Cook Time: 2 hours | Servings: 2

Ingredients:

1 pound sea bream, about 1-inch thick, cleaned

1 cup of extra virgin olive oil

1 lemon, juiced

1 tbsp sugar

1 tbsp dried rosemary

½ tbsp dried oregano

2 garlic cloves, crushed

½ cup white wine

1 tsp sea salt

Directions:

Combine olive oil with lemon juice, sugar, rosemary, oregano, crushed garlic, wine, and salt in a large bowl. Submerge fish in this mixture and marinate for one hour in the refrigerator. Remove from the refrigerator and drain but reserve the liquid for serving. Place fillets in a large vacuum-sealable bag and seal. Cook en Sous Vide for 40 minutes at 122 F. Drizzle the remaining marinade over fillets and serve.

Salmon & Kale Salad with Avocado

Prep + Cook Time: 1 hour | Servings: 3

Ingredients:

1 pound skinless salmon fillet

Salt and black pepper to taste

½ organic lemon, juiced

1 tbsp olive oil

1 cup kale leaves, shredded

½ cup roasted carrots, sliced

½ ripe avocado, cut into small cubes

1 tbsp fresh dill

1 tbsp fresh parsley leaves

Directions:

Season the fillet with salt and pepper on both sides and place in a large vacuum-sealable bag. Seal the bag and cook en sous vide for 40 minutes at 122 F. Remove the salmon from a water bath and set aside.

Whisk together the lemon juice, a pinch of salt and black pepper in a mixing bowl and gradually add in olive oil while whisking constantly. Add the shredded kale and toss to evenly coat with vinaigrette. Add in the roasted carrots, avocados, dill, and parsley. Gently toss to combine. Transfer to a serving bowl and serve with salmon on top.

Gingery Salmon

Prep + Cook Time: 45 minutes | Servings: 4

Ingredients:

4 salmon filets, with skin

2 tsp sesame oil

1 ½ olive oil

2 tbsp ginger, grated

2 tbsp sugar

Directions:

Make a water bath, place Sous Vide in it, and set to 124F. Season salmon with salt and pepper. Place the remaining listed ingredient in a bowl and mix.

Place salmon and sugar mixture into two vacuum-sealable bags, release air by the water displacement method, seal and submerge the bag in the water bath. Set the timer for 30 minutes.

Once the timer has stopped, remove and unseal the bag. Place a skillet over medium heat, place a piece of parchment paper at the bottom and preheat. Add the salmon, skin down, and sear for 1 minute each. Serve with a side of buttered broccoli.

Mussels in Fresh Lime Juice

Prep + Cook Time: 40 minutes | Servings: 2

Ingredients:

1 pound fresh mussels, debearded

1 medium-sized onion, peeled and finely chopped

Garlic cloves, crushed

½ cup freshly squeezed lime juice

¼ cup fresh parsley, finely chopped

1 tbsp rosemary, finely chopped

2 tbsp olive oil

Directions:

Place mussels along with lime juice, garlic, onion, parsley, rosemary, and olive oil in a large vacuum-sealable bag. Cook en Sous Vide for 30 minutes at 122 F. Serve with green salad.

Herb-Marinated Tuna Steaks

Prep + Cook Time: 1 hour 25 minutes | Servings: 5

Ingredients:

2 pounds tuna steaks, about 1-inch thick

1 tsp dried thyme, ground

1 tsp fresh basil, finely chopped

¼ cup finely chopped shallots

2 tbsp fresh parsley, finely chopped

1 tbsp fresh dill, finely chopped

1 tsp freshly grated lemon zest

½ cup sesame seeds

4 tbsp olive oil

Salt and black pepper to taste

Directions:

Wash the tuna fillets under cold running water and pat dry with a kitchen paper. Set aside.

In a large bowl, combine thyme, basil, shallots, parsley, dill, oil, salt, and pepper. Mix until well incorporated and then soak the steaks in this marinade. Coat well and refrigerate for 30 minutes.

Place the steaks in a large vacuum-sealable bag along with marinade. Press the bag to remove the air and seal the lid. Cook en Sous Vide for 40 minutes at 131 degree.

Remove the steaks from the bag and transfer to a kitchen paper. Gently pat dry and remove the herbs. Preheat a skillet over high temperature. Roll the steaks in sesame seeds and transfer to the skillet. Cook for 1 minute on each side and remove from the heat.

Crabmeat Patties

Prep + Cook Time: 65 minutes | Servings: 4

Ingredients:

1 pound lump crab meat

1 cup red onions, finely chopped

½ cup red bell peppers, finely chopped

2 tbsp chili pepper, finely chopped

1 tbsp celery leaves, finely chopped

1 tbsp parsley leaves, finely chopped

½ tsp tarragon, finely chopped

Salt and black pepper to taster

4 tbsp olive oil

2 tbsp almond flour

3 eggs, beaten

Directions:

Heat 2 tablespoons of olive oil in a skillet and add onions. Stir-fry until translucent and add chopped red bell peppers and chili pepper. Cook for 5 minutes, stirring constantly.

Transfer to a large bowl. Add crab meat, celery, parsley, tarragon, salt, pepper, almond flour, and eggs. Stir well and mold the mixture into 2-inches diameter patties. Gently divide patties between 2 vacuum-sealable bags and seal them. Cook in sous vide for 40 minutes at 122 F.

Heat the remaining olive oil in a non-stick grill pan, over high heat. Remove the patties from the water bath and transfer to a skillet. Briefly, brown on both sides for 3-4 minutes and serve.

Chili Smelts

Prep + Cook Time: 1 hour 15 minutes | Servings: 5

Ingredients:

1 pound fresh smelts

½ cup lemon juice

3 garlic cloves, crushed

1 tsp salt

1 cup extra virgin olive oil

2 tbsp fresh dill, finely chopped

1 tbsp chives, minced

1 tbsp chili pepper, ground

Directions:

Rinse smelts under cold running water and drain. Set aside.

In a large bowl, combine olive oil with lemon juice, crushed garlic, sea salt, finely chopped dill, minced chives, and chili pepper. Place smelts into this mixture and cover. Refrigerate for 20 minutes.

Remove from the refrigerator and place in a large vacuum-sealable bag along with the marinade. Cook in sous vide for 40 minutes at 104 F. Remove from the water bath and drain but reserve the liquid.

Heat a large skillet over medium heat. Add smelts and briefly cook, for 3-4 minutes, turning them over. Remove from the heat and transfer to a serving plate. Drizzle with marinade and serve immediately.

Marinated Catfish Fillets

Prep + Cook Time: 1 hour 20 minutes | Servings: 3

Ingredients:

1 pound catfish fillet

½ cup lemon juice

½ cup parsley leaves, finely chopped

2 garlic cloves, crushed

1 cup onions, finely chopped

1 tbsp fresh dill, finely chopped

1 tbsp fresh rosemary leaves, finely chopped

2 cups freshly squeezed apple juice

2 tbsp Dijon mustard

1 cup extra virgin olive oil

Directions:

In a large bowl, combine lemon juice, parsley leaves, crushed garlic, finely chopped onions, fresh dill, rosemary, apple juice, mustard, and olive oil. Whisk together until well incorporated. Submerge fillets in this mixture and cover with a tight lid. Refrigerate for 30 minutes.

Remove from the refrigerator and place in 2 vacuum-sealable bags. Seal and cook in sous vide for 40 minutes at 122 F. Remove and drain; reserve the liquid. Serve drizzled with its own liquid.

Parsley Prawns with Lemon

Prep + Cook Time: 35 minutes | Servings: 4

Ingredients:

12 large prawns, peeled and deveined

1 tsp salt

1 tsp sugar

3 tsp olive oil

1 bay leaf

1 sprig parsley, chopped

2 tbsp lemon zest

1 tbsp lemon juice

Directions:

Make a water bath, place Sous Vide in it, and set to 156 F. In a bowl, add prawns, salt, and sugar, mix and let it sit for 15 minutes. Place prawns, bay leaf, olive oil, and lemon zest in a vacuum-sealable bag. Release air by the water displacement method and seal. Submerge in bath and cook for 10 minutes.Once the timer has stopped, remove and unseal the bag. Dish prawns and drizzle with lemon juice.

Sous Vide Halibut

Prep + Cook Time: 1 hour 20 minutes | Servings: 4

Ingredients:

1 pound halibut fillets

3 tbsp olive oil

¼ cup of shallots, finely chopped

1 tsp freshly grated lemon zest

½ tsp dried thyme, ground

1 tbsp fresh parsley, finely chopped

1 tsp fresh dill, finely chopped

Salt and black pepper to taste

Directions:

Wash the fish under cold running water and pat dry with a kitchen paper. Cut into thin slices generously sprinkle with salt and pepper. Place in a large vacuum-sealable bag and add two tablespoons of olive oil. Season with shallots, thyme, parsley, dill, salt, and pepper.

Press the bag to remove the air and seal the lid. Shake the bag to coat all fillets with spices and refrigerate for 30 minutes before cooking. Cook in sous vide for 40 minutes at 131 F.

Remove the bag from water and set aside to cool for a while. Place on a kitchen paper and drain. Remove the herbs.

Preheat the remaining oil in a large skillet over high temperature. Add fillets and cook for 2 minutes. Flip the fillets and cook for about 35-40 seconds and then remove from the heat. Transfer the fish again to a paper towel and remove excessive fat. Serve immediately.

Lemon Butter Sole

Prep + Cook Time: 45 minutes | Servings: 3

Ingredients:

3 sole filets

1 ½ tbsp unsalted butter

¼ cup lemon juice

½ tsp lemon zest

Lemon pepper to taste

1 sprig parsley for garnishing

Directions:

Make a water bath, place Sous Vide in it, and set to 132 F. Pat dry the sole and place in 3 separate vacuum-sealable bag. Release air by the water displacement method and seal the bags. Submerge in the water bath and set the timer for 30 minutes.

Place a small pan over medium heat, add in butter. Once it has melted remove from the heat. Add lemon juice and lemon zest and stir.

Once the timer has stopped, remove and unseal the bag. Transfer the sole filets to serving plates, drizzle butter sauce over and garnish with parsley. Serve with a side of steam green vegetables.

Basil Cod Stew

Prep + Cook Time: 50 minutes | Servings: 4

Ingredients:

1 pound cod fillet

1 cup fire-roasted tomatoes

1 tbsp basil, dried

1 cup fish stock

2 tbsp tomato paste

3 celery stalks, finely chopped

1 carrot, sliced

¼ cup olive oil

1 onion, finely chopped

½ cup button mushrooms

Directions:

Heat olive oil in a large skillet, over medium heat. Add celery, onions, and carrot. Stir-fry for 10 minutes. Remove from the heat and transfer to a vacuum-sealable bag along with other ingredients. Cook in sous vide for 40 minutes at 122 F.

Easy Tilapia

Prep + Cook Time: 1 hour 10 minutes | Servings: 3

Ingredients

3 (4 oz) tilapia filets

3 tbsp butter

1 tbsp apple cider vinegar

Salt and black pepper to taste

Directions:

Make a water bath, place Sous Vide in it, and set to 124 F. Season the tilapia with pepper and salt and place in a vacuum-sealable bag. Release air by the water displacement method and seal the bag. Submerge it in the water bath and set the timer for 1 hour.

Once the timer has stopped, remove and unseal the bag. Put a skillet over medium heat and add butter and vinegar. Simmer and stir continually to reduce vinegar by half. Add the tilapia and sear slightly. Season with salt and pepper as desired. Serve with a side of buttered vegetables.

Salmon with Asparagus

Prep + Cook Time: 3 hours 15 minutes | Servings: 6

Ingredients:

1 pound wild salmon fillet

1 tbsp olive oil

1 tbsp dried oregano

12 medium asparagus spears

4 white onion rings

1 tbsp fresh parsley

Salt and black pepper to taste

Directions:

Season the fillet with oregano, salt, and pepper on both sides and lightly brush with olive oil.

Place in a large vacuum-sealable along with other ingredients. Combine all spices in a mixing bowl. Rub the mixture evenly on both sides of the steak and place in a large vacuum-sealable bag. Seal the bag and cook in sous vide for 3 hours at 136 F.

Curry Mackerel

Prep + Cook Time: 55 minutes | Servings: 3

Ingredients:

3 mackerel filets, heads removed

3 tbsp curry paste

1 tbsp olive oil

Salt and black pepper to taste

Directions:

Make a water bath, place Sous Vide in it, and set to 120 F. Season the mackerel with pepper and salt and place in a vacuum-sealable bag. Release air by the water displacement method, seal and submerge it in the water bath, and set the timer for 40 minutes.

Once the timer has stopped, remove and unseal the bag. Set a skillet over medium heat, add olive oil. Coat the mackerel with the curry powder (do not pat the mackerel dry)

Once it has heated, add the mackerel and sear until golden brown.Serve with a side of steamed green leafy vegetables.

Rosemary Squid

Prep + Cook Time: 1 hour and 15 minutes | Servings: 3

Ingredients:

1 pound fresh squid, whole

½ cup extra virgin olive oil

1 tbsp of pink Himalayan salt

1 tbsp of dried rosemary

3 garlic cloves, crushed

3 cherry tomatoes, halved

Directions:

Thoroughly rinse each squid under the running water. Using a sharp paring knife, remove the heads and clean each squid.

In a large bowl, combine olive oil with salt, dried rosemary, cherry tomatoes, and crushed garlic. Submerge squid in this mixture and refrigerate for 1 hour. Then remove and drain. Place squid and cherry tomatoes in a large vacuum-sealable bag. Cook en sous vide for one hour at 136 F.

Fried Lemon Shrimps

Prep + Cook Time: 50 minutes | Servings: 3

Ingredients:

1 pound shrimps, peeled and deveined

3 tbsp olive oil

½ cup freshly squeezed lemon juice

1 garlic clove, crushed

1 tsp fresh rosemary, crushed

1 tsp sea salt

Directions:

Combine olive oil with lemon juice, crushed garlic, rosemary, and salt. Using a kitchen brush, spread the mixture over each shrimp and place in a large vacuum-sealable bag. Cook in sous vide for 40 minutes at 104 F.

Octopus Grill

Prep + Cook Time: 5 hours 20 minutes | Servings: 3

Ingredients:

½ lb medium octopus tentacles, blanched

Salt and black pepper to taste

3 tsp + 3 tbsp olive oil

2 tsp dried oregano

2 sprigs fresh parsley, chopped

Ice for an ice bath

Directions:

Make a water bath, place Sous Vide in it, and set to 171 F.

Place octopus, salt, 3 teaspoons of olive oil, and pepper in a vacuum-sealable bag. Release air by the water displacement method, seal and submerge the bag in water bath. Set timer for 5 hours.

Once the timer has stopped, remove the bag and cover in an ice bath. Set aside. Preheat a grill.

Once the grill is hot, transfer the octopus to a plate, add 3 tablespoons of olive oil and massage. Grill octopus to char nicely on each side. Dish octopus and garnish with parsley and oregano. Serve with a sweet, spicy dip.

Wild Salmon Steaks

Prep + Cook Time: 1 hour 25 minutes | Servings: 4

Ingredients:

2 pounds wild salmon steaks

3 garlic cloves, crushed

1 tbsp fresh rosemary, finely chopped

1 tbsp freshly squeezed lemon juice

1 tbsp freshly squeezed orange juice

1 tsp orange zest

1 tsp pink Himalayan salt

1 cup fish stock

Directions:

Combine orange juice with lemon juice, rosemary, garlic, orange zest, and salt. Brush the mixture over each steak and refrigerate for 20 minutes. Transfer to a large vacuum-sealable bag and add fish stock. Seal the bag and cook in sous vide for 50 minutes at 131 F.

Preheat a large, non-stick grill pan. Remove the steaks from vacuum-sealable bag and grill for 3 minutes on each side, until lightly charred.

Tilapia Stew

Prep + Cook Time: 65 minutes | Servings: 3

Ingredients:

1 pound tilapia fillets

½ cup onions, finely chopped

1 cup carrots, finely chopped

½ cup cilantro leaves, finely chopped

3 garlic cloves, finely chopped

1 cup green bell peppers, finely chopped

1 tsp Italian seasoning mix

1 tsp cayenne pepper

½ tsp chili pepper

1 cup fresh tomato juice

Salt and black pepper to taste

3 tbsp olive oil

Directions:

Heat olive oil over medium heat. Add chopped onions and stir-fry until translucent.

Now add bell pepper, carrots, garlic, cilantro, Italian seasoning mix, cayenne pepper, chili pepper, salt, and black pepper. Give it a good stir and cook for ten more minutes.

Remove from the heat and transfer to a large vacuum-sealable bag along with tomato juice and tilapia fillets. Cook in sous vide for 50 minutes at 122 F. Remove from the water bath and serve.

Buttery Cockles with Peppercorns

Prep + Cook Time: 1 hour 30 minutes | Servings: 2

Ingredients:

4 oz canned cockles

¼ cup dry white wine

1 diced celery stalk

1 diced parsnip

1 quartered shallot

1 bay leaf

1 tbsp black peppercorns

1 tbsp olive oil

8 tbsp butter, room temperature

1 tbsp minced fresh parsley

2 garlic cloves, minced

Salt to taste

1 tsp freshly cracked black pepper

¼ cup panko breadcrumbs

1 baguette, sliced

Directions:

Prepare a water bath and place the Sous Vide in it. Set to 154 F. Place the cockles, shallots, celery, parsnip, wine, peppercorns, olive oil and bay leaf in a vacuum-sealable bag. Release air by the water displacement method, seal and submerge the bag in the water bath. Cook for 60 minutes.

Using a blender, pour the butter, parsley, salt, garlic and ground pepper. Mix at medium speed until combined. Put the mixture into a plastic bag and roll it. Move into the fridge and allow chilling.

Once the timer has stopped, remove the snail and veggies. Discard the cooking juices. Heat a skillet over high heat. Top the cockles with butter, sprinkle some breadcrumbs over and cook for 3 minutes until melted. Serve with warm baguette slices.

Cilantro Trout

Prep + Cook Time: 60 minutes | Servings: 4

Ingredients:

2 pounds trout, 4 pieces

5 garlic cloves

1 tbsp sea salt

4 tbsp olive oil

1 cup cilantro leaves, finely chopped

2 tbsp rosemary, finely chopped

¼ cup freshly squeezed lemon juice

Directions:

Clean and rinse well the fish. Pat dry with a kitchen paper and rub with salt. Combine garlic with olive oil, cilantro, rosemary, and lemon juice. Use the mixture to fill each fish. Place in a separate vacuum-sealable bags and seal. Cook en Sous Vide for 45 minutes at 131 F.

Squid Rings

Prep + Cook Time: 1 hour 25 minutes | Servings: 3

Ingredients:

2 cups squid rings

1 tbsp fresh rosemary

Salt and black pepper to taste

½ cup olive oil

Directions:

Combine squid rings with rosemary, salt, pepper, and olive oil in a large clean plastic bag. Seal the bag and shake a couple of times to coat well. Transfer to a large vacuum-sealable and seal the bag. Cook in sous vide for 1 hour and 10 minutes at 131 F. Remove from the water bath and serve.

Chili Shrimp & Avocado Salad

Prep + Cook Time: 45 minutes | Servings: 4

Ingredients:

1 chopped red onion

Juice of 2 limes

1 tsp olive oil

¼ tsp sea salt

⅛ tsp white pepper

1 pound raw shrimp, peeled and deveined

1 diced tomato

1 diced avocado

1 green chili pepper, seeded and diced

1 tbsp chopped cilantro

Directions:

Prepare a water bath and place the Sous Vide in it. Set to 148 F.

Place the lime juice, red onion, sea salt, white pepper, olive oil, and shrimp in a vacuum-sealable bag. Release air by the water displacement method, seal and submerge the bag in the water bath. Cook for 24 minutes.

Once the timer has stopped, remove the bag and transfer to an ice-water bath for 10 minutes. In a bowl, combine the tomato, avocado, green chili pepper, and cilantro. Pour the bag contents on top.

Buttery Red Snapper with Citrus Saffron Sauce

Prep + Cook Time: 55 minutes | Servings: 4

Ingredients

4 pieces cleaned red snapper

2 tbsp butter

Salt and black pepper to taste

<u>For Citrus Sauce</u>

1 lemon

1 grapefruit

1 lime

3 oranges

1 tsp Dijon mustard

2 tbsp canola oil

1 yellow onion

1 diced zucchini

1 tsp saffron threads

1 tsp diced chili pepper

1 tbsp sugar

3 cups fish stock

3 tbsp chopped cilantro

Directions

Prepare a water bath and place the Sous Vide in it. Set to 132 F. Season the snapper fillets with salt and pepper and place in a vacuum-sealable bag. Release air by the water displacement method, seal and submerge the bag in the water bath. Cook for 30 minutes.

Peel the fruits and chop in cubes. Heat oil in a skillet over medium heat and put the onion and zucchini. Sauté for 2-3 minutes. Add the fruits, saffron, pepper, mustard and sugar. Cook for 1 minute more. Stir the fish stock and simmer for 10 minutes. Garnish with cilantro, and set aside. Once the timer has stopped, remove the fish and transfer to a plate. Glaze with citrus-saffron sauce and serve.

Sesame-Crusted Cod Fillet

Prep + Cook Time: 45 minutes | Servings: 2

Ingredients

1 large cod fillet

2 tbsp sesame paste

1½ tbsp brown sugar

2 tbsp fish sauce

2 tbsp butter

Sesame seeds

Directions

Prepare a water bath and place the Sous Vide in it. Set to 131 F.

Soak cod with the brown sugar, sesame paste and fish sauce mixture. Place in a vacuum-sealable bag. Release air by the water displacement method, seal and submerge the bag in the water bath. Cook for 30 minutes. Melt butter in a skillet over medium heat.

Once the timer has stopped, remove the cod and transfer to the skillet and sear for 1 minute. Serve onto a platter. Pour cooking juices into the skillet and cook until reduced. Add 1 tbsp of butter and mix. Top cod with the sauce and garnish with sesame seeds. Serve with rice.

Creamy Salmon with Spinach & Mustard Sauce

Prep + Cook Time: 55 minutes | Servings: 2

Ingredients

4 skinless salmon fillets

1 large bunch of spinach

½ cup Dijon mustard

1 cup heavy cream

1 cup half-and-half cream

1 tbsp lemon juice

Salt and black pepper to taste

Directions

Prepare a water bath and place the Sous Vide in it. Set to 115 F. Place the salmon seasoned with salt in a vacuum-sealable bag. Release air by the water displacement method, seal and submerge the bag in the water bath. Cook for 45 minutes.

Heat a pot over medium heat and cook spinach until softened. Lower the heat and pour in lemon juice, pepper and salt. Keep cooking. Heat a saucepan over medium heat and combine the half-and-half cream and Dijon mustard. Lower the heat and cook. Season with salt and pepper. Once the timer has stopped, remove the salmon and transfer to a plate. Druzzle with sauce. Serve with spinach.

Paprika Scallops with Fresh Salad

Prep + Cook Time: 55 minutes | Servings: 4

Ingredients

1 pound scallops

1 tsp garlic powder

½ tsp onion powder

½ tsp paprika

¼ tsp cayenne pepper

Salt and black pepper to taste

<u>Salad</u>

3 cups corn kernels

½ pint halved cherry tomatoes

1 diced red bell pepper

2 tbsp chopped fresh parsley

<u>Dressing</u>

1 tbsp fresh basil

1 quartered lemon

Directions

Prepare a water bath and place the Sous Vide in it. Set to 122 F.

Place the scallops in a vacuum-sealable bag. Season with salt and pepper. In a bowl, combine the garlic powder, paprika, onion powder, and cayenne pepper. Pour inside. Release air by the water displacement method, seal and submerge the bag in the water bath. Cook for 30 minutes.

Meanwhile, preheat the oven to 400 F. In a baking tray, put the corn kernels and red pepper. Sprinkle olive oil and season with salt and pepper. Cook for 5-10 minutes. Transfer to a bowl and mix with parsley. In a bowl, combined well the dressing ingredients and pour over corn kernels.

Once the timer has stopped, remove the bag and transfer to a hot skillet. Sear for 2 minutes each side. Serve on a platter, the scallops, and salad. Garnish with basil and lemon wedge.

Saucy Scallops with Mango

Prep + Cook Time: 50 minutes | Servings: 4

Ingredients

1 pound large scallops

1 tbsp butter

Sauce

1 tbsp lemon juice

2 tbsp olive oil

Garnish

1 tbsp lime zest

1 tbsp orange zest

1 cup diced mango

1 thinly sliced Serrano pepper

2 tbsp chopped mint leaves

Directions

Place the scallops in a vacuum-sealable bag. Season with salt and pepper. Allow chilling in the fridge all night. Prepare a water bath and place the Sous Vide in it. Set to 122 F. Release air by the water displacement method, seal and submerge the bag in the water bath. Cook for 15-35 minutes.

Heat a skillet over medium heat. In a bowl, combine well the sauce ingredients. Once the timer has stopped, remove the scallops and transfer to the skillet and sear until browned. Serve in a plate. Sprinkle the sauce and add the garnish ingredients.

Leek & Shrimp with Mustard Vinaigrette

Prep + Cook Time: 1 hour 20 minutes | Servings: 4

Ingredients

6 leeks

5 tbsp olive oil

Salt and black pepper to taste

1 shallot, minced

1 tbsp rice vinegar

1 tsp Dijon mustard

1/3 pound cooked bay shrimp

Chopped fresh parsley

Directions

Prepare a water bath and place the Sous Vide in it. Set to 183 F.

Cut the top of the leeks and remove the bottom parts. Wash them in cold water and sprinkle with 1 tbsp of olive oil. Season with salt and pepper. Place in a vacuum-sealable bag. Release air by the water displacement method, seal and submerge the bag in the water bath. Cook for 1 hour.

Meanwhile, for the vinaigrette, in a bowl combine the shallot, Dijon mustard, vinegar, and 1/4 cup of olive oil. Season with salt and pepper. Once the timer has stopped, remove the bag and transfer to an ice-water bath. Allow cooling. Put the leeks in 4 plates and season with salt. Add the shrimp and drizzle with vinaigrette. Garnish with parsley.

Coconut Shrimp Soup

Prep + Cook Time: 55 minutes | Servings: 6

Ingredients

8 large raw shrimp, peeled and de-veined

1 tbsp butter

Salt and black pepper to taste

For Soup

1 pound zucchini

4 tbsp lime juice

2 yellow onions, chopped

1-2 small red chilis, finely chopped

1 stem of lemongrass, white part only, chopped

1 tsp shrimp paste

1 tsp sugar

1½ cups coconut milk

1 tsp tamarind paste

1 cup water

½ cup coconut cream

1 tbsp fish sauce

2 tbsp fresh basil, chopped

Directions

Prepare a water bath and place the Sous Vide in it. Set to 142 F. Place the shrimp and butter in a vacuum-sealable bag. Season with salt and pepper. Release air by the water displacement method, seal and submerge the bag in the water bath. Cook for 15-35 minutes.

Meanwhile, peel the zucchini and discard the seeds. Chop in cubes. In a food processor, add the onion, lemongrass, chili, shrimp paste, sugar, and 1/2 cup of coconut milk. Blend until purée.

Heat a casserole over lower heat and combine the onion mixture, remaining coconut milk, tamarind paste and water. Add in zucchini and cook for 10 minutes.

Once the timer has stopped, remove the shrimp and transfer to the soup. Whisk the coconut cream, lime juice and basil. Serve in soup bowls.

Honey Salmon with Soba Noodles

Prep + Cook Time: 40 minutes | Servings: 4

Ingredients

Salmon

6 oz salmon fillets, skin-on

Salt and black pepper to taste

1 tsp sesame oil

1 cup olive oil

1 tbsp fresh ginger, grated

2 tbsp honey

Sesame Soba

4 oz dry soba noodles

1 tbsp grapeseed oil

2 garlic cloves, chopped

½ cauliflower head

3 tbsp tahini

1 tsp sesame oil

2 tsp olive oil

¼ juiced lime

1 sliced stalk green onion

¼ cup cilantro, roughly chopped

1 tsp toasted poppy seeds

Lime wedges for garnish

Sesame seeds for garnish

2 tbsp cilantro, chopped

Directions

Prepare a water bath and place the Sous Vide in it. Set to 123 F. Season the salmon with salt and pepper. In a bowl, combine sesame oil, olive oil, ginger and honey. Place the salmon and mixture in a vacuum-sealable bag. Shake well. Release air by the water displacement method, seal and submerge the bag in the water bath. Cook for 20 minutes.

Meanwhile, prepare the soba noodles. Heat grapeseed oil in a skillet over high heat and stir-fry cauliflower and garlic for 6-8 minutes. In a bowl, combine well the tahini, olive oil, sesame oil, lime juice, cilantro, green onions and toasted sesame seeds. Drain the noodles and add to the cauliflower.

Heat a skillet over high heat. Cover with baking paper sheet. Once the timer has stopped, remove the salmon and transfer to the skillet. Sear for 1 minute. Serve the noodles in two bowls and add in salmon. Garnish with lime wedges, poppy seeds, and cilantro.

Gourmet Lobster with Mayonnaise

Prep + Cook Time: 40 minutes | Servings: 2

Ingredients

2 lobster tails

1 tbsp butter

2 sweet onions, chopped

3 tbsp mayonnaise

Salt to taste

A pinch of black pepper

2 tsp lemon juice

Directions

Prepare a water bath and place the Sous Vide in it. Set to 138 F.

Heat water in a casserole over high heat, until boiling. Open the lobster tails shells and immerse into the water. Cook for 90 seconds. Transfer to an ice-water bath. Allow cooling for 5 minutes. Crack the shells and remove the tails.

Place the tails with butter in a vacuum-sealable bag. Release air by the water displacement method, seal and submerge the bag in the water bath. Cook for 25 minutes.

Once the timer has stopped, remove the tails and pat dry. Seat aside. Allow chilling for 30 minutes. In a bowl, combine the mayonnaise, sweet onions, pepper, and lemon juice. Chop the tails, add to the mayonnaise mixture, and stir well. Serve with toasted bread.

Party Shrimp Cocktail

Prep + Cook Time: 40 minutes | Servings: 2

Ingredients

1 pound shrimp, peeled and deveined

Salt and black pepper to taste

4 tbsp fresh dill, chopped

1 tbsp butter

4 tbsp mayonnaise

2 tbsp green onions, minced

2 tsp freshly squeezed lemon juice

2 tsp tomato puree

1 tbsp tabasco sauce

4 oblong dinner rolls

8 leaves of lettuce

½ lemon, sliced into wedges

Directions

Prepare a water bath and place the Sous Vide in it. Set to 149 F. For the seasoning, combine well the mayonnaise, green onions, lemon juice, tomato puree, and Tabasco sauce. Season with salt and pepper.

Place the shrimp and seasoning in a vacuum-sealable bag. Add 1 tbsp of dill and 1/2 tbsp of butter in each pack. Release air by the water displacement method, seal and submerge the bag in the water bath. Cook for 15 minutes.

Preheat the oven over 400 F. and cook the dinner rolls for 15 minutes. Once the timer has stopped, remove the bag and drain. Put the shrimp in a bowl with the dressing and mix well. Serve on top of the lettuce rolls with lemon.

Herby Lemon Salmon

Prep + Cook Time: 45 minutes | Servings: 2

Ingredients

2 skinless salmon fillets

Salt and black pepper to taste

¾ cup extra virgin olive oil

1 shallot, sliced into thin rings

1 tbsp basil leaves, lightly chopped

1 tsp allspice

3 oz mixed greens

1 lemon

Directions

Prepare a water bath and place the Sous Vide in it. Set to 128 F.

Place the salmon and season with salt and pepper in a vacuum-sealable bag. Add in shallot rings, olive oil, allspice, and basil. Release air by the water displacement method, seal and submerge the bag in the water bath. Cook for 25 minutes.

Once the timer has stopped, remove the bag and transfer the salmon to a plate. Mix the cooking juices with some lemon juice and top salmon fillets. Serve.

Savory Buttery Lobster Tails

Prep + Cook Time: 1 hour 10 minutes | Servings: 2

Ingredients

8 tbsp butter

2 lobster tails, shells removed

2 sprigs fresh tarragon

2 tbsp sage

Salt to taste

Lemon wedges

Directions

Prepare a water bath and place the Sous Vide in it. Set to 134 F.

Place the lobster tails, butter, salt, sage and tarragon in a vacuum-sealable bag. Release air by the water displacement method, seal and submerge the bag in the water bath. Cook for 60 minutes.

Once the timer has stopped, remove the bag and transfer the lobster to a plate. Sprinkle butter on top. Garnish with lemon wedges.

Thai Salmon with Cauliflower & Egg Noodles

Prep + Cook Time: 55 minutes | Servings: 2

Ingredients

2 skin-on salmon fillets

Salt and black pepper to taste

1 tbsp olive oil

4½ tbsp soy sauce

2 tbsp minced fresh ginger

2 thinly sliced Thai Chilis

6 tbsp sesame oil

4 oz prepared egg noodles

6 oz cooked cauliflower florets

5 tsp sesame seeds

Directions

Prepare a water bath and place the Sous Vide in it. Set to 149 F. Prepare a baking tray lined with aluminium foil and put the salmon, season with salt and pepper and cover with another aluminium sheet. Bake in the oven for 30 minutes.

Remove the baked salmon to a vacuum-sealable bag. Release air by the water displacement method, seal and submerge the bag in the water bath. Cook for 8 minutes.

In a bowl, mix ginger, chilis, 4 tbsp of soy sauce, and 4 tbsp of sesame oil. Once the timer has stopped, remove the bag and transfer the salmon to a noodle bowl. Garnish with toasted seeds and salmon skin. Sprinkle with the ginger-chillies sauce and serve.

Light Sea Bass with Dill

Prep + Cook Time: 35 minutes | Servings: 3

Ingredients

1 pound Chilean sea bass, skinless

1 tbsp olive oil

Salt and black pepper to taste

1 tbsp dill

Directions

Prepare a water bath and place the Sous Vide in it. Set to 134 F. Season the sea bass with salt and pepper and place in a vacuum-sealable bag. Add the dill and olive oil. Release air by the water displacement method, seal and submerge the bag in the water bath. Cook for 30 minutes. Once the timer has stopped, remove the bag and transfer the sea bass to a plate.

Sweet Chili Shrimp Stir-Fry

Prep + Cook Time: 40 minutes | Servings: 6

Ingredients

1½ pound shrimp

3 dried red chilis

1 tbsp grated ginger

6 garlic cloves, smashed

2 tbsp champagne wine

1 tbsp soy sauce

2 tsp sugar

½ tsp cornstarch

3 green onions, chopped

Directions

Prepare a water bath and place the Sous Vide in it. Set to 135 F.

Combine the ginger, garlic cloves, chilis, champagne wine, sugar, soy sauce, and cornstarch. Place the peeled shrimp with the mixture in a vacuum-sealable bag. Release air by the water displacement method, seal and submerge in the water bath. Cook for 30 minutes.

Place green onions in a skillet over medium heat. Add in oil and cook for 20 seconds. Once the timer has stopped, remove the cooked shrimp and transfer to a bowl. Garnish with onion. Serve with rice.

Fruity Thai Shrimp

Prep + Cook Time: 25 minutes | Servings: 4

Ingredients

2 pounds shrimp, peeled and deveined

4 pieces peeled and shredded papaya

2 shallots, sliced

¾ cup cherry tomatoes, halved

2 tbsp basil, chopped

¼ cup toasted dry pan peanuts

Thai Dressing

¼ cup lime juice

6 tbsp sugar

5 tbsp fish sauce

4 garlic cloves

4 small red chili

Directions

Prepare a water bath and place the Sous Vide in it. Set to 135 F. Place the shrimp in a vacuum-sealable bag. Release air by the water displacement method, seal and submerge the bag in the water bath. Cook for 15 minutes. Combine well in a bowl the lime juice, fish sauce and sugar. Mash the garlic and chilis. Add to the dressing mixture.

Once the timer has stopped, remove the shrimp from the bag and transfer to a bowl. Add the papaya, Thain basil, shallots, tomato and peanuts. Glaze with the dressing.

Dublin-Style Lemon Shrimp Dish

Prep + Cook Time: 1 hour 15 minutes | Servings: 4

Ingredients

4 tbsp butter

2 tbsp lime juice

2 cloves fresh garlic, minced

1 tsp fresh lime zest

Salt and black pepper to taste

1 pound jumbo shrimp, peeled and de-veined

½ cup of panko breadcrumbs

1 tbsp fresh parsley, minced

Directions

Prepare a water bath and place the Sous Vide in it. Set to 135 F.

Heat 3 tbsp of butter in a skillet over medium heat and add in lime juice, salt, pepper, garlic, and zest. Allow cooling for 5 minutes. Place the shrimp and mixture in a vacuum-sealable bag. Release air by the water displacement method, seal and submerge the bag in the water bath. Cook for 30 minutes.

Meanwhile, heat butter in a pan over medium and toast the panko breadcrumbs. Once the timer has stopped, remove the shrimp and transfer to a hot pot over high heat and cook with the cooking juices. Serve in 4 soup bowls and top with the breadcrumbs.

Juicy Scallops with Chili Garlic Sauce

Prep + Cook Time: 75 minutes | Servings: 2

Ingredients

2 tbsp yellow curry powder

1 tbsp tomato paste

½ cup coconut cream

1 tsp chili garlic sauce

1 tbsp lemon juice

6 scallops

Cooked brown rice, for serving

Fresh cilantro, chopped

Directions

Prepare a water bath and place the Sous Vide in it. Set to 134 F.

Combine the coconut cream, tomato paste, curry powder, lime juice, and chili-garlic sauce. Place the mixture with the scallops in a vacuum-sealable bag. Release air by the water displacement method, seal and submerge the bag in the water bath. Cook for 60 minutes.

Once the timer has stopped, remove the bag and transfer to a plate. Serve the brown rice and top with the scallops. Garnish with cilantro.

Curry Shrimp with Noodles

Prep + Cook Time: 25 minutes | Servings: 2

Ingredients

1 pound shrimp, tail-on

8 oz vermicelli noodles, cooked and drained

1 tsp rice wine

1 tsp curry powder

1 tbsp soy sauce

1 green onion, sliced

2 tbsp vegetable oil

Directions

Prepare a water bath and place the Sous Vide in it. Set to 149 F. Place the shrimp in a vacuum-sealable bag. Release air by the water displacement method, seal and submerge the bag in the water bath. Cook for 15 minutes.

Heat oil in a pan over medium heat and add in rice wine, curry powder and soy sauce. Mix well and combine the noodles. Once the timer has stopped, remove the shrimp and transfer to the noodle mix. Garnish with green onion.

Savory Creamy Cod with Parsley

Prep + Cook Time: 40 minutes | Servings: 6

Ingredients

For Cod

6 cod fillets

Salt to taste

1 tbsp olive oil

3 sprigs fresh parsley

For Sauce

1 cup white wine

1 cup half-and-half cream

1 finely chopped white onion

2 tbsp dill, chopped

2 tsp black peppercorns

Directions

Prepare a water bath and place the Sous Vide in it. Set to 148 F.

Place seasoned with salt cod fillets in vacuum-sealable bags. Add olive oil and parsley. Release air by the water displacement method, seal and submerge the bag in the water bath. Cook for 30 minutes.

Heat a saucepan over medium heat, add in wine, onion, black peppercorns and cook until reduced. Stir in half-and-half cream until thickened. Once the timer has stopped, plate the fish and drizzle with sauce.

French Pot de Rillettes with Salmon

Prep + Cook Time: 2 hours 30 minutes | Servings: 2

Ingredients

½ pound salmon fillets, skin removed

1 tsp sea salt

6 tbsp butter

1 onion, chopped

1 garlic clove, minced

1 tbsp lime juice

Directions

Prepare a water bath and place the Sous Vide in it. Set to 130 F. Place the salmon, unsalted butter, sea salt, garlic cloves, onion and lemon juice in a vacuum-sealable bag. Release air by the water displacement method, seal and submerge the bag in the water bath. Cook for 20 minutes.

Once the timer has stopped, remove the salmon and transfer into 8 small bowls. Season with cooking juices. Allow chilling in the fridge for 2 hours. Serve with toast bread slices.

Sage Salmon with Coconut Potato Mash

Prep + Cook Time: 1 hour 30 minutes | Servings: 2

Ingredients

2 salmon fillets, skin-on

2 tbsp olive oil

2 sprigs sage

4 garlic cloves

3 potatoes, pelled and chopped

¼ cup coconut milk

1 bunch rainbow chard

1 tbsp grated ginger

1 tbsp soy sauce

Sea salt to taste

Directions

Prepare a water bath and place the Sous Vide in it. Set to 122 F. Place salmon, sage, garlic, and olive oil in a vacuum-sealable bag. Release air by the water displacement method, seal and submerge the bag in the water bath. Cook for 1 hour.

Heat an oven to 375 F. Brush the potatoes with oil and bake for 45 minutes. Transfer potatoes to a blender and add in coconut milk. Season with salt and pepper. Blend for 3 minutes, until smooth.

Heat olive oil in a skillet over medium heat and sauté ginger, chard and soy sauce.

Once the timer has stopped, remove the salmon and transfer to a hot pan. Sear for 2 minutes. Transfer to a plate, add the potato mash, and top with char to serve.

Dill Baby Octopus Bowl

Prep + Cook Time: 60 minutes | Servings: 4

Ingredients

1 pound baby octopus

1 tbsp olive oil

1 tbsp freshly squeezed lemon juice

Salt and black pepper to taste

1 tbsp dill

Directions

Prepare a water bath and place the Sous Vide in it. Set to 134 F. Place the octopus in a vacuum-sealable bag. Release air by the water displacement method, seal and submerge the bag in the water bath. Cook for 50 minutes. Once the timer has stopped, remove the octopus and pat dry. Mix the octopus with some olive oil and lemon juice. Season with salt, pepper and dill.

Salted Salmon in Hollandaise Sauce

Prep + Cook Time: 1 hour 50 minutes | Servings: 4

Ingredients

4 salmon fillets

Salt to taste

Hollandaise Sauce

4 tbsp butter

1 egg yolk

1 tsp lemon juice

1 tsp water

½ diced shallot

A pinch of paprika

Directions

Season the salmon with salt. Allow chilling for 30 minutes. Prepare a water bath and place the Sous Vide in it. Set to 148 F. Place all the sauce ingredients in a vacuum-sealable bag. Release air by the water displacement method, seal and submerge the bag in the water bath. Cook for 45 minutes.

Once the timer has stopped, remove the bag. Set aside. Lower the temperature of the Sous Vide to 120 F and place salmon in a vacuum-sealable bag. Release air by the water displacement method, seal and submerge the bag in the water bath. Cook for 30 minutes. Transfer the sauce to a blender and mix until light yellow. Once the timer has stopped, remove the salmon and pat dry. Serve topped with the sauce.

Amazing Lemon Salmon with Basil

Prep + Cook Time: 35 minutes | Servings: 4

Ingredients

2 pounds salmon

2 tbsp olive oil

1 tbsp chopped basil

Zest of 1 lemon

Juice of 1 lemon

¼ tsp garlic powder

Sea salt and black pepper to taste

Directions

Prepare a water bath and place the Sous Vide in it. Set to 115 F. Place the salmon in a vacuum-sealable bag. Release air by the water displacement method, seal and submerge the bag in the water bath. Cook for 30 minutes.

Meanwhile, in a bowl combine well the pepper, salt, basil, lemon juice, and garlic powder until emulsified. Once the timer has stopped, remove the salmon and transfer to a plate. Reserve the cooking juices. Heat olive oil in a pan over high heat and sauté the garlic slices. Set aside the garlic. Put the salmon in the pan and cook for 3 minutes until golden. Plate and top with the garlic slices.

Egg Bites with Salmon & Asparagus

Prep + Cook Time: 70 minutes | Servings: 6

Ingredients

6 whole eggs

¼ cup crème fraiche

¼ cup goat cheese

4 spears asparagus

2 oz smoked salmon

2 oz chèvre cheese

½ oz minced shallot

2 tsp chopped, fresh dill

Salt and black pepper to taste

Directions

Prepare a water bath and place the Sous Vide in it. Set to 172 F. Blend the eggs, crème fraiche, goat cheese and salt. Diced the asparagus and add to the mix with the shallots. Cut salmon and add to the bowl as well. Add the dill. Combine well.

Add the egg and salmon mixture into 6 jars. Add 1/6 chevre into the jars, seal and submerge the jars in the water bath. Cook for 60 minutes. Once the timer has stopped, remove the jars and top with salt.

Garlicky Mustard Shrimp

Prep + Cook Time: 2 hours 45 minutes | Servings: 2

Ingredients

½ tsp yellow mustard seeds

¼ tsp celery seeds

½ tsp red pepper flakes

½ tsp coriander seeds

½ tsp fennel seeds

¾ cup olive oil

½ cup freshly squeezed lemon juice

4 tbsp rice vinegar

Salt and black pepper to taste

1 bay leaves

1 tbsp Old Bay Seasoning

2 garlic cloves, very thinly sliced

1 pound deveined shrimp

½ yellow onion, cut into thin slices

Directions

Prepare a water bath and place the Sous Vide in it. Set to 149 F.

Heat a saucepan over medium heat and toast the mustard seeds, red pepper flakes, celery, fennel and coriander seeds. Cook until pop. Set aside and allow cooling.

In a canning jar pour the olive oil, lemon juice, toasted spices, black pepper, rice vinegar, bay leaves, garlic cloves and seasoning. Seal and submerge the jars in the water bath. Cook for 30 minutes.

Once the timer has stopped, remove the jars and allow cooling for 5 minutes. Transfer to an ice-water bath for cooling. Put in the fridge for 2 hours before serving.

Yummy Cheesy Lobster Risotto

Prep + Cook Time: 55 minutes | Servings: 4

Ingredients

1 tall lobster, shell removed

Salt and black pepper to taste

6 tbsp butter

2½ cups chicken stock

¾ cup Arborio rice

2 tbsp red wine

¼ cup grated Grana Padano cheese

2 minced chives

Directions

Prepare a water bath and place the Sous Vide in it. Set to 138 F. Season the lobster with salt and pepper and place in a vacuum-sealable bag with 3 tbsp of butter. Release air by the water displacement method, seal and submerge the bag in the water bath. Cook for 25 minutes.

Heat 3 tbsp of butter in a skillet over medium heat and cook the rice. Stir in 1/4 cup of chicken stock. Keep cooking until the stock evaporated. Add 1/4 cup of chicken stock more. Repeat the process for 15 minutes until the rice is creamy.

Once the timer has stopped, remove the lobster and chop in bites. Add the lobster to the rice. Stir the remaining chicken stock and red wine. Cook until liquid is absorbed. Top with Grana Padano cheese and season with salt and pepper. Garnish with chives and more cheese.

CPSIA information can be obtained
at www.ICGtesting.com
Printed in the USA
LVHW010152210622
721700LV00011B/421

9 781804 508008